Primary Care
Pediatric
Otolaryngology

Second Edition

Primary Care
Pediatric
Otolaryngology

Second Edition

William P. Potsic, M.D.
Professor of Otorhinolaryngology and Head-Neck Surgery
University of Pennsylvania School of Medicine
Director, Division of Otolaryngology and Human Communication
The Children's Hospital of Philadelphia
Philadelphia, Pennsylvania

Steven D. Handler, M.D.
Associate Professor of Otorhinolaryngology and Head-Neck Surgery
University of Pennsylvania School of Medicine
Associate Director, Division of Otolaryngology and Human Communication
The Children's Hospital of Philadelphia
Philadelphia, Pennsylvania

Ralph F. Wetmore, M.D.
Associate Professor of Otorhinolaryngology and Head-Neck Surgery
University of Pennsylvania School of Medicine
Division of Otolaryngology and Human Communication
The Children's Hospital of Philadelphia
Philadelphia, Pennsylvania

Patrick S. Pasquariello, Jr., M.D.
Professor of Pediatrics
University of Pennsylvania School of Medicine
Director, Diagnostic Center
The Children's Hospital of Philadelphia
Philadelphia, Pennsylvania

1995 **J. Michael Ryan Publishing, Inc.** • Andover, New Jersey

Primary Care Pediatric Otolaryngology
William P. Potsic, Steven D. Handler, Ralph F. Wetmore, Patrick S. Pasquariello, Jr.

Library of Congress Catalog Card Number   95-67933

J. Michael Ryan Publishing, Inc.
24 Crescent Drive North
Andover, New Jersey 07821

Important Note: Medicine is an ever-changing science. Research and clinical experience are continually broadening our knowledge. Insofar as this book mentions any dosage or applications, readers may rest assured that the authors have made every effort to ensure that such references are strictly in accordance with the current state of knowledge and standards of practice at the time of the publication of this book. Nevertheless, it is every reader's responsibility to carefully examine the manufacturer's literature accompanying pharmaceuticals to verify whether the dosage schedules recommended therein or contraindications cited differ from the statements made in this book. Readers are reminded that such examination is particularly important with drugs that are either rarely used or have been newly released on the market.

Some of the product names, patents, and registered designs referred to in this book are in fact registered trademarks or proprietary names even though specific reference to this fact is not always made in the text. Therefore, the appearance of a name without designation as proprietary is not to be construed as a representation that it is in the public domain.

Printed in the United States of America.

ISBN 1-887064-00-1

Preface to the Second Edition

Reader response to the first edition of *Primary Care Pediatric Otolaryngology* has been very gratifying. This text has proved to be a valuable resource to primary care physicians in their management of children.

We have incorporated the comments and advice of our readers in this new edition. We have updated the book and we have broadened its scope with the addition of Ralph Wetmore, a pediatric otolaryngologist, and Patrick Pasquariello, a primary care physician at The Children's Hospital of Philadelphia.

We hope that this second edition meets your expectations and needs in the managment of children with otolaryngologic disorders.

William P. Potsic, M.D.
Steven D. Handler, M.D.
Ralph F. Wetmore, M.D.
Patrick S. Pasquariello, Jr., M.D.

Preface to the First Edition

Primary Care Pediatric Otolaryngololgy is a concise, practical guide to the diagnosis and management of head and neck disorders in children, the most commonly encountered pediatric complaints in primary care practice. Our goal has been to present essential information in a convenient format and to omit the nonessential, establishing clear criteria for diagnosis, for treatment, and for referral. Our desire to make the book easy to use dictated the editorial focus, organization of the text, selection of illustrations and references, and design and layout.

Organization of the text by anatomic area makes it possible to incorporate the essentials of anatomy and physiology into each chapter. This same organization is also well suited to a thorough discussion of the conditions commonly affecting each anatomic area. We do not catalogue rare head and neck disorders, as this would interfere with our principal goals: ease of use and practical orientation. However, rare conditions that can mimic more common disorders are described; we provide criteria for making a timely differential diagnosis and we offer practical tips on primary treatment.

We hope this guide will contribute to improved cooperation between the primary care physician and the pediatric otolaryngologist.

William P. Potsic, M.D.
Steven D. Handler, M.D.

Contents

Chapter 2

NOSE AND PARANASAL SINUSES 59

Chapter 3

ORAL CAVITY AND PHARYNX 87

Chapter 4

LARYNX AND TRACHEA 111

Chapter 5

NECK AND ASSOCIATED STRUCTURES 143

CHAPTER 1

EAR

ANATOMY

The ear can be divided into three anatomic compartments. The external or outer ear is composed of the auricle, the external auditory canal, and the lateral surface of the eardrum. The middle ear is the space between the tympanic membrane and the inner ear. The inner ear contains the vestibular apparatus and the cochlea (Fig. 1-1).

The auricle or pinna has a cartilage framework covered by skin and subcutaneous tissue. The external canal is directed posteriorly and superiorly at its lateral extent and continues in a more anterior and horizontal direction in its medial portion. The lateral two thirds of the canal consists of cartilage lined with skin containing hair follicles and cerumen glands. The medial one third is contained within the temporal bone and is lined with a very thin skin devoid of all skin appendages.

The tympanic membrane separates the middle ear from the external ear. The short and long process of the malleus are embedded in the middle (fibrous) layer of the tympanic membrane and are easily seen within the substance of the drum. The portion of the tympanic membrane below the level of the short process is the pars tensa. It has three layers, consisting of skin (outer layer), fibrous (middle layer), and mucosa (inner layer). The pars flaccida is the portion of the drum above the short process of the malleus and is de-

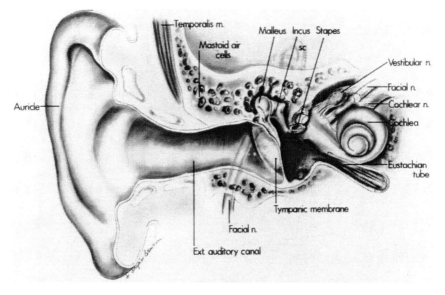

Figure 1–1. Diagram of the external, middle, and inner ear, SC = semicircular canals. (From Potsic WP, Handler SD, Wetmore RF: Ear, Nose, Throat and Mouth. In: Rudolph A (ed). Pediatrics. 19th ed. Norwalk, CT, Appleton & Lange, 1991.)

void of a fibrous layer. The tympanic membrane is surrounded by a fibrous ring of tissue (the annulus), which anchors it firmly to the temporal bone (Fig. 1-2).

The middle ear cleft is an air-filled space surrounded by bone and the tympanic membrane. It communicates with the mastoid air-cell system posteriorly and with the nasopharynx through the eustachian tube anteriorly. The surface of the middle ear, as well as that of the mastoid air cells and eustachian tube, is covered with ciliated respiratory epithelium. Secretory and ciliated cells are distributed in an organized fashion that facilitates mucociliary transport from the mastoid to the eustachian tube and into the nasopharynx.

In the middle ear cleft, the ossicles bridge the gap between the tympanic membrane and the inner ear. The malleus, incus, and stapes are connected by true articular joints and are supported by fibrous bands and mucosal folds in the middle ear space. The tensor tympani and stapedius muscles originate in the bony wall of the middle ear and attach by tendons to the malleus and stapes, respectively. The tensor tympani muscle is innervated by the fifth cranial nerve, and the stapedius muscle is innervated by the seventh cranial nerve. The chorda tympani nerve passes across the medial surface of the eardrum in the posterior superior quadrant and is the afferent nerve for taste for the anterior two thirds of the tongue on each side. On the medial wall of the middle ear cleft, the facial nerve passes horizontally above the oval window, where the footplate of the stapes is located. The facial nerve is usually covered by a thin layer of bone, but portions of the bony canal may be absent. Posterior to the oval window, the facial nerve turns inferiorly, exiting at the stylomastoid foramen. The round window is covered by a membrane and lies in a niche directly inferior to the oval window. The first of the two three-quarter turns of the cochlea produces a bony projection between the round and oval window called the promontory.

The inner ear consists of the vestibular labyrinth and the cochlea. These hollowed-out spaces are surrounded by dense bone in the petrous portion of the temporal bone. The membranous labyrinth, the various compartment of which are filled with specialized fluids (perilymph and endolymph), is contained within these bony spaces.

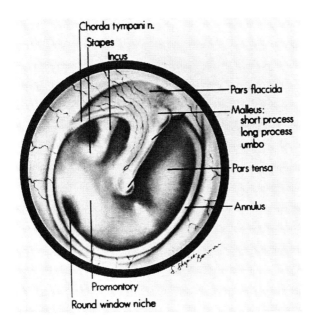

Figure 1–2. Otoscopic view of normal right tympanic membrane and middle ear structures. (From Potsic WP, Handler SD, Wetmore RF: Ear, Nose, Throat and Mouth. In: Rudolph A (ed). Pediatrics. 19th ed. Norwalk, CT, Appleton & Lange, 1991.)

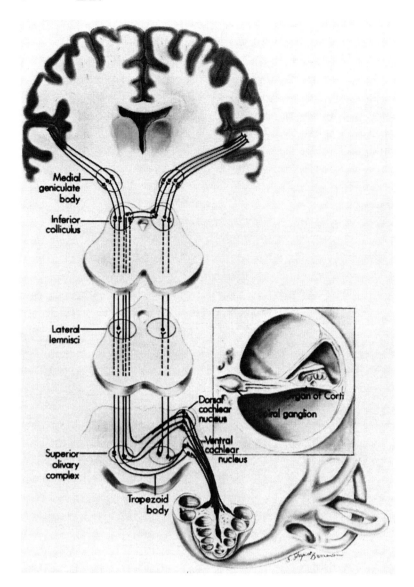

Figure 1–3. Diagrammatic representation of the auditory pathway.

The dilated end of each semicircular canal contains the vestibular sense organ (the crista ampullaris), which is responsive to acceleration changes in head position. The utricle and saccule each have a sense organ (a macula) that responds to gravitational forces. Each vestibular sense organ consists of specialized responsive cells (hair cells) and accompanying supporting cells. The cochlea is tubular and has two three-quarter turns. The organ of Corti, the sense organ of hearing, is suspended within the cochlea by the basilar membrane and is bathed in perilymph and endolymph. The organ of Corti consists of hair cells and supporting cells.

The hair cells of the cochlea and vestibular labyrinth send their sensory information through a cortex network of neural conditions to the cerebral cortex (Fig. 1-3).

PHYSIOLOGY

External Ear

The auricle helps collect incoming sound and the external ear canal directs it to the tympanic membrane. This process enhances the directional properties of sound; with phase differences between the two ears, it provides a mechanism for sound localization.

Middle Ear

The tympanic membrane and ossicles couple the outer ear to the inner ear. Surface area differences between the tympanic membrane and oval window (17:1) produce a mechanical advantage in the transmission of sound. The tensor tympani and stapedius muscles stiffen the ossicular chain as they contract in response to loud sounds. This process is thought to be a protective mechanism to avoid noise-induced injury to the inner ear.

The secretory elements of the middle ear create a mucus blanket. Ciliary action results in movement of the mucus blanket from the mastoid and middle ear through the eustachian tube to the nasopharynx. This active transport process is referred to as the mucociliary transport system. Ciliary function, as well as the mechanical properties of the mucus, can affect the rate of mucus transport. Middle ear mucus has an optimal viscosity and elasticity for transport. If mucus is thinner or thicker than optimal, it will not be transported efficiently. The mucociliary transport system also clears bacteria and cellular debris from the mastoid and middle ear. This clearing mechanism, along with secretory immunoglobulins and lysozymes, helps prevent and resolve middle ear infections.

The eustachian tube is the only connection between the middle ear and nasopharynx. In addition to clearing secretions, it permits equalization of pressure between the middle ear and the atmosphere as it opens during swallowing or yawning.

Inner Ear

Oscillation of the stapes footplate within the oval window transfers sound into the inner ear. Fluid waves travel from the basal turn of the cochlea to the apex, displacing the basilar membrane. Maximum displacement occurs at a point along the basilar membrane specific for each frequency: high frequencies in the basal turn and low frequencies at the apex. Vibration of the basilar membrane causes bending of the hairs of the sensory cells in the organ of Corti and produces an action potential that is transmitted along the auditory pathway to the cerebral cortex. Coding of information about intensity (loudness) and frequency (pitch) in the action potential occurs throughout the auditory pathway.

The vestibular apparatus responds to the flow of fluid within the vestibular labyrinth upon changes in head position or movement. Movement of endolymph causes hair cell depolarization and produces an action potential that is transmitted to the vestibular cortex. The semicircular canals respond to changes in acceleration (head movement). The utricle and saccule respond to gravity or to linear acceleration (position). These vestibular sensors, together with proprioception and visual orientation, maintain balance and regulate body position.

METHODS OF EXAMINATION

Physical Examination

Proper equipment is essential to a good ear examination and should include a brightly illuminated pneumatic otoscope, several specula of various sizes, and a wax loop or curette. An illuminated headlight or a 100 watt bulb and head mirror should be available as well. A small otologic forceps can also be of great assistance.

The examination should begin with inspection of the shape of the pinna and skin on the front and back of the ear. The scalp, face, and neck around the ear should also be inspected. The opening of the external canal (external meatus) should be examined first with the naked eye. The meatus can be fully opened by pulling the pinna into a posterior-superior direction with one hand and the tragus forward by traction on the skin in

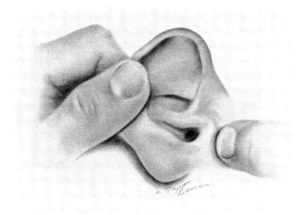

Figure 1–4. The external meatus is opened by pulling the auricle in the posterior-superior direction and by placing traction on the skin immediately in front of the tragus.

front of the ear with the other hand (Fig 1-4).

The more medial aspect of the ear canal should then be inspected with a brightly illuminated otoscope, using the largest speculum that will fit in the meatus without being painful. If wax if found blocking the canal and impeding visualization of the tympanic membrane, it should be removed or pushed aside along the walls of the canal. In the neonate, vernix caseosum frequently may block the ear canal and must also be cleared to permit visualization of the tympanic membrane. Unless wax is impairing visualization of the tympanic membrane or is blocking the canal completely, causing a hearing loss, it need not be removed.

If wax or debris is impairing visualization of the tympanic membrane, the wax curette is advanced, if possible, along a portion of the canal at which the cerumen is not adherent. The mass of wax is then rolled out by withdrawing the curette while applying constant gentle pressure against the wax until it is brought out into the speculum or out of the meatus. Care should be taken to avoid scraping the ear canal, which would cause intense pain or bleeding, or both. If the wax is in the medial one third of the canal against the canal against the tympanic membrane or is too firmly adherent to the canal to be removed painlessly with a curette, irrigation of the ear canal with body temperature water will usually flush the wax out. An ear syringe, a 20 ml syringe with a flexible intravenous catheter tip, or a Water-Pik® can be used to direct the stream of water along the posterior wall of the ear canal. With repeated irrigation, the wax is flushed to the

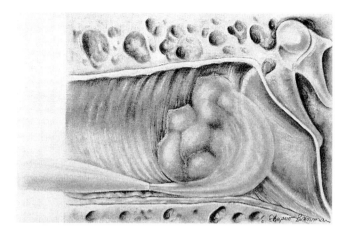

Figure 1–5. Water is directed along the floor and posterior wall of the ear canal to flush out the wax.

meatus (Fig. 1-5). Irrigation of the ear canal, however, should not be done if there is a known perforation of the tympanic membrane, a tympanostomy tube in place, or blood in the canal that might indicate a perforation of the tympanic membrane. If clearing of the wax if not urgent, antibiotic eardrops or a solution of one half peroxide and one half water, or a commercially available product (Debrox®, Murine Drops for the Ear®) can be used. Four or five drops of any of these solutions in the ear canal twice daily for four to five days will soften firm wax and facilitate clearing by irrigation.

After cleaning the external canal of wax and debris, the tympanic membrane and middle ear contents may be examined. Often the tympanic membrane can be seen by direct vision utilizing a headlight or head mirror even without an ear speculum. However, a brightly illuminated otoscope with a large speculum provides a good seal in the canal for pneumatic otoscopic examination, as well as a wide magnified field of vision. The ear canal should be straightened by traction on the pinna as the speculum is introduced and advanced. In the easily collapsible neonatal ear, the canal can be gently dilated with pressure applied through a pneumatic otoscope as the speculum is advanced to visualize the tympanic membrane. The drum should be examined and its thickness, vascularity, and contour assessed. All aspects of the tympanic membrane, including the pars flaccida, must be seen to complete the examination.

The mobility of the tympanic membrane should be assessed in each patient by applying gentle intermittent pressure to the external ear canal with a pneumatic bulb or by blowing through a rubber tube connected to the otoscope head. The posterior-superior quadrant of the tympanic membrane is the portion of the drum with the widest excursions, making it the easiest portion of the drum to assess for mobility. The neonatal ear canal is very pliable; careful observation is required to avoid confusing ear canal distention with movement of the tympanic membrane. If a slight leak of air is present around the speculum, blowing harder will compensate for the leak and permit movement of the tympanic membrane. Normal ranges of mobility can be learned only by repeated examination of each patient seen in the office.

Much has been said about the light reflex as an indicator of a normal tympanic membrane. The light reflex represents the light reflected from the surface of the tympanic membrane directly back to the examiner's eye. It usually appears in the anterior-inferior quadrant of the tympanic membrane and indicates that part of the drum that is perpendicular to the line of vision. However, the reflex can be altered by rotating the light source or by moving the patient's head. The light reflex can also be present in a grossly abnormal ear, such as one with a perforated tympanic membrane. For these reasons, we consider the light reflex an unreliable sign and of little value in the otoscopic examination.

The normal tympanic membrane is translucent, permitting the contents of the middle ear space to be seen through the drum. A complete examination of the ear should include an inspection of the middle ear through the translucent tympanic membrane. Fluid of varying colors and air-fluid interfaces may be seen, as well as the white shadow of the ossicles and the promontory in most cases. On the medial surface of the drum, the chorda tympani nerve may be seen crossing along the posterior-superior quadrant (*see* Fig 1-2). In the posterior-inferior quadrant of the middle ear, the dome of the jugular bulb occasionally can be seen as a blue shadow. Rarely, the carotid artery is visible in the anterior-inferior quadrant.

Hearing Assessment

Although hearing screening tests can detect significant hearing impairments, they do not provide sufficient information for diagnosis or rehabilitation. Evaluation by an audiologist is warranted when hearing impairment is suspected. Certified audiologists have, at a minimum, a master's degree in their field and a year of supervised postgraduate clinical experience. Since the testing of young children involves special procedures and equipment, it may be preferable to refer to an audiologist with extensive pediatric experience.

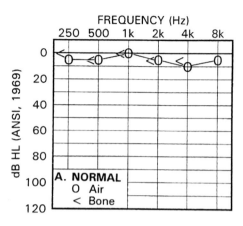

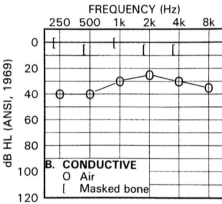

Figure 1–6. Audiograms. Results are shown only for the right ear. Thresholds are plotted as decibels hearing level (dB HL); 0 dB HL is normal hearing and higher numbers reflect hearing loss. In normal hearing (**A**), thresholds are at or near 0 dB. In conductive hearing impairment (**B**), thresholds are elevated for air conduction (sound delivered through earphones), but not for bone conduction in which vibrations are transmitted through the skull to the cochlea, bypassing the conductive apparatus of the middle ear. Here, masking was employed; white noise was delivered to the left ear during bone-conduction testing of the right, so that the patient would not detect the stimulus in the left cochlea. In sensorineural hearing impairment (**C**) the impairment is in the cochlea (or rarely in the auditory nerve) so that thresholds are elevated for both air and bone conduction.

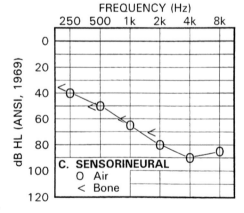

Children of any age, including newborns, can be tested by a variety of methods. Older children are most commonly assessed by conventional audiometry in which sensitivity to electronically controlled tones and speech are measured. Considerable information can be elicited from younger children by observing conditioned or reflexive responses to sound, or engaging them in play activities that encourage responding to their test stimuli. Brain-stem response audiometry permits identification of hearing impairment and estimation of its severity in infants or other children who cannot be tested behaviorally. If there is a concern only about middle ear status, impedance audiometry (tympanometry) directly measures the mechanical properties of the tympanic membrane and middle ear that affect sound transmission into the cochlea. Finally, there are tests of central auditory processing. The use of these tests in children is controversial,however, and generally should be reserved for children older than eight years of age. In the case of the child with a suspected auditory processing problem, it may be more productive to ensure normal peripheral hearing and to seek a psychological, speech/language and development evaluation.

Hearing tests are available for children of all ages and rehabilitation can be instituted in the first months of life; therefore, there is no rationale for postponing an evaluation when hearing impairment is suspected. Parental suspicion of hearing loss in an infant is an indication for audiological evaluation, even if the infant appears to respond to loud sounds.

Conventional Audiometry

In the conventional hearing test, the patient's sensitivity to tones of various frequencies or pitches is determined and graphed as an audiogram (Fig 1-6). The audiologist may determine sensitivity to bone-conducted stimuli delivered by a vibrator held against the head, as well as by earphones. Since the sound is transmitted through the skull directly to the cochlea, any impairment of the conductive apparatus is bypassed. Comparison of air- and bone-conduction sensitivity indicates whether the hearing impairment is sensorineural, conductive, or mixed. In addition to this pure-tone audiogram, the audiologist may employ other tests if additional information is needed for diagnostic or rehabilitation purposes.

Impedance Audiometry

Impedance audiometry, also known as tympanometry, is a technique that has proven very useful in evaluating middle ear status in children. The

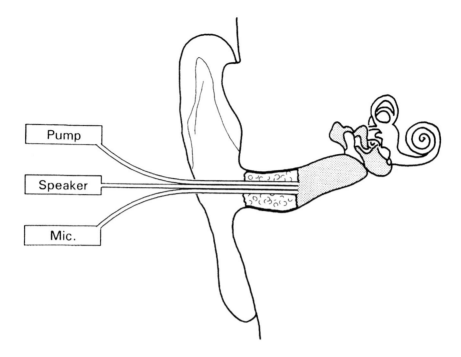

Figure 1–7. Schematic diagram of impedance audiometer. A small speaker delivers a tone to the ear canal, and the tone's intensity is measured by the microphone. A low intensity corresponds to high middle ear compliance – most of the sound energy is transmitted into the middle and inner ear. The pump varies the pressure in the ear canal; the peak compliance, illustrated in Figure 1–8A and C, appears when the applied pressure balances the pressure in the middle ear.

test does not require a voluntary response from the child, although it is difficult to perform if the child is moving or screaming. The instrument determines the compliance of the ear drum, the ease with which sound is transmitted through it. A tone is delivered into the ear canal and its intensity is measured. A low intensity implies that the sound energy has been transmitted efficiently into the middle ear (Fig 1-7). The tympanogram (Fig 1-8) shows how the compliance varies as pressure in the ear canal is varied. The peak appears when the applied pressure in the canal matches the pressure in the middle ear. In a resolving middle ear effusion, there may be some air in the middle ear, but at a reduced pressure, so that the peak is shifted to the left. If the middle ear is immobile at all applied pressures, and the tympanogram is flat.

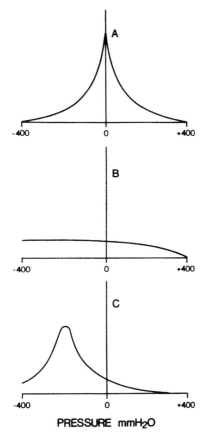

Figure 1–8. Tympanograms. (**A**) Type A: normal. (**B**) Type B: flat (usually associated with middle ear effusion). (**C**) Type C: negative middle ear pressure (eustachian tube dysfunction).

Although impedance audiometry provides information about the mechanics of the ossicles and tympanic membrane, it is not diagnostic in itself. It is a useful screening device, differentiating normal middle ear function from abnormal, and as an adjutant to otoscopy.

Brain-stem Response Audiometry

The most definitive test of auditory function, in infancy and in patients who cannot cooperate for pure tone testing, is based on the auditory brain-stem response (ABR), also known as brain-stem auditory evoked response (BAER). If the cochlea is stimulated by an abrupt stimulus such as a click, a pattern of waves can be recorded from the auditory nerve and the brain-stem auditory

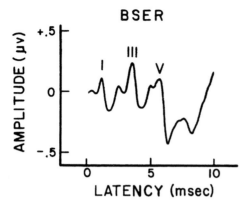

Figure 1–9. Normal brainstem evoked response elicited by 80 dB (nHL) click.

pathways (Fig. 1-9). This response can be recorded with EEG electrodes even with stimuli that are barely audible.

To avoid interference from muscle activity, the child must be asleep for the test. Young infants can be tested in natural sleep, but sedation is usually employed for older infants and young children. Although ABR testing may be offered by EEG laboratories for neurologic evaluation, it is important that the tests of auditory function be performed by audiologists or those familiar with the protocols and analyses used for auditory testing, since they differ from those used in neurodiagnosis.

Vestibular Testing

Vestibular testing in younger children, beyond behavioral observation of gait, body movement, and eye movement, is difficult because vestibular tests are unpleasant and may cause vertigo, nausea, and vomiting. In older children, the most useful test is electronystagmography. This test records eye movements using electrodes taped on the face and can be done with the patient's eyes closed. Since each eye has a corneoretinal potential, movements are easily recorded for a defined time period and displayed on a strip recorder. Spontaneous and induced nystagmus (rhythmic alternating eye movement with a fast and slow component) are detected as signs of vestibular function and dysfunction. While the slow component of the nystagmus represents the labyrinthine response to stimulation, the direction of the nystagmus is named after the fast component, or correcting eye movement.

The labyrinths can be activated by head positioning or by spinning the patient in a chair. Spinning and positioning, however, stimulate both labyrinths simultaneously and, thus, may not detect a unilateral problem.

Caloric stimulation can be performed on each labyrinth separately using cold or warm water in the ear canal. For office testing without a strip recorder, the nystagmus response can be observed after 20 ml of cold tap water is flushed slowly into the ear canal with a syringe. The temperature gradient produces convection currents in the endolymph and stimulates the labyrinth. Cooling the ear canal should cause a conjugate horizontal nystagmus toward the opposite ear. Warming should cause nystagmus to the same side. This is easily remembered by the mnemonic COWS (cold-opposite-warm-same). An injured or diseased labyrinth will display a reduced or absent nystagmus response compared with the other side.

Radiologic Examination

Standard mastoid radiographs are of limited value in the evaluation of ear disease. Computed tomography (CT) with one millimeter sections through the temporal bones provides fine bony and soft tissue detail. CT is preferable to magnetic resonance imaging (MR) for the evaluation of bony structures, such as the temporal bone. MR is useful in the patient who has suffered an intracranial complication of otitis media, such as brain abscess.

Facial Nerve Evaluation

The diagnosis and adequate treatment of facial nerve paralysis require definition of the portion of the nerve involved. Central facial paralysis causes paralysis only of the lower half of the face on the involved side, as the upper face receives bilateral innervation from the motor cortex.

Peripheral facial paralysis involves both the upper and lower face on the involved side. Lesions of the facial nerve can be localized by an understanding of the function and distribution of its branches. At three different levels along the course of the nerve in the temporal bone, a branch of the facial nerve with an individual function exits the main trunk of the nerve. The greater superficial petrosal nerve supplies the lacrimal gland and leaves the facial nerve trunk at the geniculate ganglion to regulate tear production. In the posterior-superior portion of the middle ear, the nerve to the stapedius muscle exits. The chorda tympani leaves the main trunk near the stylomastoid foramen to supply taste to the anterior two thirds of the tongue (Fig 1-10.) The site of the injury to the facial nerve can therefore be determined by testing lacrimation, the stapedius reflex (by tympanometry), and taste on the anterior portion of the tongue. For example, a lesion in the vertical position of the nerve just above the stylo-

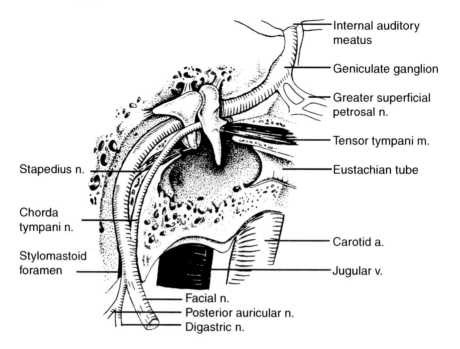

Internal auditory meatus

Geniculate ganglion

Greater superficial petrosal n.

Tensor tympani m.

Eustachian tube

Carotid a.

Jugular v.

Stapedius n.

Chorda tympani n.

Stylomastoid foramen

Facial n.

Posterior auricular n.

Digastric n.

Figure 1–10. Course of the facial nerve inside temporal bone (tympanic membrane removed).

mastoid foramen will be associated with good lacrimation and a stapedius reflex, but absent taste on the anterior two thirds of the tongue. Neuronal degeneration may be detected at three to four days after facial nerve injury but requires specialized techniques such as facial nerve electrical testing. Electromyography is clinically useful to detect fibrillation potentials from denervated muscle which occur two to three weeks after injury to the nerve.

COMMON COMPLAINTS

Ear Pain

Ear pain may be caused by an ear disorder or a condition distant from the ear (nonotogenic otalgia) (Table 1-1). Nonotogenic ear pain may represent referred pain from anywhere in the head and neck area (neuralgia) or may be psychogenic in origin. The complaint of ear pain may be communicated to the parent or examiner in many different ways. Newborn infants may not demonstrate any ear-specific behavior and may just be irritable. Prelingual children may also exhibit irritability, poor sleep habits, and may pull at their ears. Older children are generally able to verbalize that their ear hurts.

Ear pain is usually caused by an inflammatory process in the ear such as *acute otitis media* or *external otitis*. Acute otitis media causes a deep, boring and persistent pain that is not exacerbated by pulling on or touching the pinna. Children frequently say their ear hurts when they feel the fluctuations of pressure in the middle ear with *secretory otitis media*. *Herpes zoster oticus* presents with vesicles on the pinna and is associated with severe pain. Tumors of the external ear canal and middle ear may also cause pain in the involved ear.

The most perplexing situation involves the complaint of ear pain in a normal-appearing ear. The most likely cause of such pain is a separate process in an area innervated by a nerve that also supplies the ear, called *referred otalgia*. Neuralgias of many of the nerves supplying the head and neck region can cause typical pain in their primary distribution, as well as referred ear pain. The sensory innervation of the ear consists of four cranial and two cervical nerves. Referred pain may be caused by an inflammatory process anywhere in the distribution of these nerves.

TABLE 1-1 Causes of Earache

Otogenic
   Infection
      Viral otitis media
      Bacterial otitis media
      External otitis
Nonotogenic
   Regional pain
      Temporomandibular joint pain
      Parotitis
      Preauricular cervical adenitis
   Referred pain
      C1 and C2 cervical spine disease
      Cranial nerve
         V (toothache)
         VII (anterior tongue lesions)
         IX and X (pharyngeal or laryngeal inflammation)
Psychogenic pain

The most common source of referred ear pain is via the *fifth cranial nerve* and is usually of dental origin. In young children, erupting teeth may cause ear discomfort. In older children, fractured or infected teeth may be sources of pain. In adolescents, impacted molars are a frequent source of ear pain. Other causes of pain referred along the fifth nerve include ulcerations of the oral mucosa (aphthous ulcers), sinusitis, and sialadenitis of the submandibular or parotid gland. While temporomandibular joint dysfunction causes pain just anterior to the ear, it can be misinterpreted as ear pain. Very rarely, intracranial lesions such as abscesses or tumors can refer pain to the ear via the middle meningeal branch of the fifth nerve.

The *ninth cranial nerve* supplies the oral pharynx, nasopharynx, and posterior third of the tongue. Inflammation in the nasopharynx (adenoids) and tonsils is a common source of referred pain. The ear pain commonly experienced after tonsillectomy or adenoidectomy tends to worsen with swallowing. Malignant tumors of the nasopharynx, such as rhabdomyosarcomas, are another possible cause of ear pain.

The *tenth cranial nerve* supplies the base of the tongue, hypopharynx, larynx, and trachea. Inflammatory lesions in these areas may cause referred pain to the ear. Vocal cord ulcers, laryngitis, tracheitis or, rarely, rheumatoid arthritis of cricoarytenoid joint may be associated with ear pain.

Ear pain via the *seventh cranial nerve* usually accompanies Bell's Palsy or herpes zoster oticus (Ramsay Hunt syndrome). The pain usually precedes the facial paralysis or skin eruption by 24 to 48 hours. Rarely, facial nerve tumors cause ear pain.

Cervical nerves C2 and *C3* supply the mastoid region and posterior pinna through the greater occipital and greater auricular nerves. Cervical spine injuries such as fractures or whiplash injuries can cause ear pain through those nerves. Arthritis, vertebral disc disease, and muscle tension are other sources of pain referred to the ear region.

When the otologic examination shows no abnormal findings, and no lesion causing referred pain can be found in the distribution of the above-discussed nerves, a psychogenic origin of pain must be considered. In these case, the area of pain usually does not fit the region of sensory supply of the four cranial or two cervical nerves that supply the ear. The child may also appear tense or depressed. One must be careful, however, when labeling ear pain as psychogenic, because a small lesion that goes undetected at the first examination may become evident at a later date. Any patient with unexplained ear pain should be referred to an otolaryngologist and a complete head and neck examination should be performed, including visualization of the nasopharynx, hypopharynx, and larynx.

Hearing Loss

Hearing loss is not a common complaint reported by children. In most cases, parents or teachers are the ones to notice the suspected impairment. In infants, subtle or vague behavioral abnormalities suggesting decreased responsiveness to sound may indicate hearing loss. Older children may have delayed language and speech development as the first sign of a hearing loss. As a child reaches four to five years of age, a hearing loss may be detected in a school screening evaluation. Hearing loss in one ear often goes undetected until school age because children with one normal ear usually do not demonstrate any obvious impairment in communicative skills.

Hearing loss may be classified as *conductive* or *sensorineural*. Conductive hearing loss is caused by an abnormality of either the ear canal, tympanic membrane, or middle ear ossicles. Sensorineural hearing loss is related to abnormalities in the inner ear or, more centrally, in the auditory pathway. Hearing impairments may be either conductive or sensorineural, or a combination of the two. Hearing loss should be further classified as persistent (stable), fluctuating, or progressive. The amount of hearing loss — mild, moderate, severe, or profound — and the frequencies affected — low, high, or both — should be determined.

The most common types of hearing loss encountered in children are *conductive* in nature. The most common cause of conductive hearing loss in children and adolescents is secretory otitis media. Fluid in the middle ear causes a conductive hearing loss that may fluctuate between a mild to moderate deficit. Acute otitis media is also a common cause of conductive hearing loss. Purulent material in the middle ear cleft interferes with sound transmission and causes a hearing loss that resolves as the infection clears. Chronic otitis media with a perforated tympanic membrane is consistently associated with a conductive hearing loss because the hole decreases the efficiency of sound transmission. Other causes of conductive hearing deficits are a cerumen-plugged ear canal, congenital anomalies of the ear canal or ossicles, and ossicular discontinuity resulting from a fracture, dislocation, or necrosis. Ossicular fixation will result in decreased sound transmission and may be caused by congenital immobility, tympanosclerosis, or otosclerosis.

Sensorineural hearing loss is most often congenital (genetic or intrauterine) and unilateral. The genetic losses are usually related to a recessive trait and may be associate with abnormalities of other organ systems. These hearing losses, usually undetected until school age unless the deficits are bilateral and/or severe, may interfere with social interaction and speech development. Sensorineural deficits may be acquired as a result of a metabolic disorder such as renal tubular acidosis or hypothyroidism but most often are caused by a viral infection of the inner ear. Mumps and measles are common causes of acquired unilateral or bilateral sensorineural hearing losses, respectively. Other etiologies of sensorineural hearing loss include exposure to ototoxic drugs, especially during the neonatal period, kernicterus, head trauma, meningitis, and tumors of, or compressing, the eighth cranial nerve.

When a hearing loss is suspected, a complete examination of the ear should be performed. If the cause is not obvious, as in secretory otitis media, an audiogram should be obtained to determine the threshold of hearing and to define the type and degree of hearing loss. With the current state of technology, no child is too young to have an accurate, reliable hearing assessment. Patients with a hearing loss of unknown cause or one that does not respond to conventional management should be referred to an otolaryngologist for further evaluation and treatment.

Ear Discharge

Any discharge from the ear, other than wax, is always abnormal. The discharge associated with otitis media or external otitis may vary from thin and watery to thick, mucopurulent, and blood-tinged. These infections are usually easily distinguished by history and examination of the ear.

Chronic otitis media (persistent perforation of the tympanic membrane and/or cholesteatoma) with infection of the middle ear mucosa causes a painless mucopurulent drainage that may be blood-tinged. The foul odor of *Pseudomonas* infection is usually present. A similar discharge may occur through a tympanostomy tube when middle ear infection is present. A rare cause of otorrhea is drainage of a first branchial cleft sinus of cyst into the external canal. This discharge is usually clear, odorless (unless the cyst becomes infected), and intermittent.

Any discharge that is unexplained or that persists after adequate therapy should initiate a referral to an otolaryngologist.

Dizziness

Vertigo or dizziness is a sense of disequilibrium or imbalance. This problem may be caused by dysfunction at any point in the vestibular-auditory pathway from the external canal to the cerebral cortex. While some children describe a feeling of spinning, or of the environment spinning, others may experience symptoms of vestibular dysfunction that may be only vague feelings of imbalance that are difficult to describe. Vertigo should be suspected in a child who is observed as frightened, clinging to a parent, and experiencing sudden and recurrent bouts of nausea or vomiting. These children are also often described as clumsy by caretakers or teachers. Older children and adolescents are usually able to describe their symptoms well if a careful history is taken.

Vertigo may be associated with abnormalities of the *external and middle ear*. Complete occlusion of the external canal by wax, a foreign body, or debris from external otitis may cause dizziness or disequilibrium. The offending material is usually pushing against part of the tympanic membrane. Removal of the occluding material relieves the symptoms completely.

Eustachian tube dysfunction with tympanic membrane retraction and/or secretory otitis media is frequently associated with a vague sensation of dizziness and disequilibrium. Acute otitis media may also cause an inflammatory response in the inner ear, resulting in dizziness.

Chronic otitis media may cause vertigo in several ways. When bacterial infection is active in the middle ear space, serous labyrinthitis or acute suppurative labyrinthitis may develop. If a cholesteatoma (skin-lined sac) is present, the process may invade the bony covering of the labyrinth and expose the labyrinthine membrane to the middle ear contents as well as to pressure changes in the atmosphere. The labyrinthine membrane may be eroded, resulting in a leak of fluid (fistula). In the presence of an exposed labyrinth or fistula, pneumatic otoscopy causes vertigo when positive or negative pressure is applied to the external ear canal.

A variety of inner ear problems will often result in vertigo. *Labyrinthitis*, either primary (measles, mumps, or other virus), or secondary to an inflammatory condition of the middle ear, is associated with severe dizziness.

Serous labyrinthitis is a sterile inflammatory process without bacterial invasion of the inner ear that resolves as the infection clears. If bacteria invades the inner ear to cause acute suppurative labyrinthitis, severe vertigo and sensorineural deafness will occur. While the hearing loss is usually permanent, the vertigo will most often decrease or disappear as the contralateral labyrinth compensates.

Leaks of perilymph from the inner ear may develop as a result from trauma (head injury, ear operations) or secondary to chronic otitis media. Straining, coughing, sneezing, or barotrauma may also precipitate a fistula by rupturing the oval or round window membrane. The onset of symptoms immediately follows the precipitating event and the vertigo is usually severe. Again, as with the exposed labyrinth that can occur in chronic otitis media, pneumatic otoscopy may exacerbate the vertigo. After the initial event, persistent (or recurrent) fluctuating dizziness and sensorineural hearing loss may occur. Labyrinthine concussion, without a fistula, secondary to head trauma may also cause persistent or intermittent vertigo.

Vestibular neuronitis gradually causes a sudden onset of vertigo that resolves over a period of several weeks. The etiology is uncertain but is thought to be viral. Hearing is usually normal.

Ménière's disease (endolymphatic hydrops) is rare in children and adolescent. It is characterized by a symptom complex of vertigo, tinnitus, and a sensation of fullness in the ear. Fluctuating sensorineural hearing loss primarily in the low frequencies is present.

Benign paroxysmal vertigo of childhood usually occurs in children between the ages of one and four years. It is characterized by the sudden onset of severe vertigo that lasts for a few minutes and recurs intermittently. The etiology is unknown, and the process resolves spontaneously. Hearing is normal both during and between attacks. Benign positional vertigo also occurs in children and adolescents. It is precipitated by an abrupt change in head position and is not associated with hearing loss. The etiology is uncertain and it usually resolves spontaneously.

Retrolabyrinthine lesions may cause vertigo as well. Eighth nerve tumors in the internal auditory canal (schwannomas) and other tumors of the cerebellopontine angle cause progressive vertigo and sensorineural hearing loss.

Central nervous system causes of dizziness are uncommon in children. Most of these are associated with focal neurologic signs, however the only presenting sign of early lesions may be vertigo. Temporal lobe seizures, tumors and inflammatory processes (meningitis or brain abscess) affecting the temporal lobe also cause vertigo. Demyelinating diseases (e.g., multiple sclerosis) may also present with dizziness. Other rare causes of dizziness are migraine, thyroid dysfunction (either hyperthyroidism or hypothyroidism), diabetes mellitus, syphilis, and hyperlipidemias.

Psychogenic dizziness should be considered in a child in whom the physical findings are inconsistent with the complaints. Often symptoms may correlate with other psychological problems, such as school avoidance.

Since the symptoms of vertigo may be associated with a serious disease process, any patient with severe or persistent dizziness should be referred to an otolaryngologist for complete evaluation and possible treatment. A complete otolaryngologic and neurologic examination and sophisticated vestibular and audiometric testing are usually required to determine the source of vestibular vertigo.

Tinnitus

Tinnitus is a persistent or intermittent noise in the ear, classified as objective (which can be heard by the examiner) and subjective (which cannot be heard by the examiner). The ability to describe the nature of the tinnitus depends on the child's age. Most often when children complain of noises in the ear, they are referring to the clicking sound or sensation of the eustachian tube opening or closing. This is most common in children with secretory otitis media. Wax or fluid in the external canal can also cause a crackling sensation. Vascular causes of tinnitus produce pulsatile tinnitus synchronous with the pulse. Middle ear tumors or normal vascular structures in the middle ear such as the jugular bulb or carotid artery may be sources of pulsatile tinnitus. Most patients have tinnitus of unknown etiology thought to be related to the cochlear dysfunction associated with sensorineural loss.

CONGENITAL MALFORMATIONS

Congenital malformations of the ear vary in severity from mild cosmetic problems, which have no effect on hearing, to severe anomalies associated with profound hearing losses. They may affect any part of the ear and auditory pathway. Often, anomalies of one part of the ear are associated with malformations in other areas of the ear and, occasionally, in other organ systems (e.g., renal, musculoskeletal).

External Ear

The most common anomalies involve the visible portion of the external ear and consist of variations in shape and position of the pinna. While most of these deformities are minor and of little significance, some require further evaluation and treatment. Prominent ears, "lop ears" or, more correctly, prominotia, occurs when the pinna protrudes laterally from the head as a result of lack of development of the antihelical fold. Although this deformity has no functional significance, its appearance may be a source of embarrassment to the child. Surgical correction (otoplasty) may be considered when the child is four or five years old. By then, the ear has reached almost adult size, making the repair easier. Thus, the deformity will have been corrected before the child has started school and is subjected to teasing from classmates. Many other minor variations in the pinna occur as well, such as irregular or incomplete auricular folds. Although these are usually of no funtional significance, cosmetic surgery may be considered depending on the severity of the deformity.

Tags of skin and subcutaneous tissue are also frequently seen in the preauricular area. Some tags contain small amounts of cartilage. These anomalies are of no functional importance but can be removed for cosmetic reasons.

Preauricular sinus or cysts are another frequently seen congenital anomaly. These skin-lined tracts are found on the face just anterior to the region where the helix and tragus meet; they are caused by failure of complete fusion of two of the six auricular hillocks. The sinus tract appears as a single pit on the skin surface but may arborize extensively and even form a cyst in the subcutaneous tissues. Preauricular sinuses are of no consequences unless they retain squamous debris to form an expanding mass or become recurrently infected. Infected preauricular sinuses should be treated with antistaphylococcal antibiotics and local heat. An infection that does not respond to this regimen may require incision and drainage to treat the inflammatory process. Once the infection has been controlled, the patient should be referred to an otolaryngologist for complete excision of the sinus and all its epithelial-lined extensions.

Severe deformity or almost total absence of the auricle is referred to as microtia, which may occur unilaterally or bilaterally. Microtia is often associated with abnormalities of the external ear canal and/or middle ear structures. Any child with microtia should have a complete otologic examination and an audiogram. If any abnormal finding are noted, referral should be made to an otolaryngologist. Cosmetic repair of the microtia may be considered when the child is four or five years old. The success of surgical correction is largely a function of the amount of deformity present. Small deformities have the best chance for normal appearance. Cases of almost complete absence of the pinna are very difficult to restore to normal contour and appearance.

The external ear canal may be deformed with or without any abnormality of the pinna. Again, any child with an anomaly of the ear canal should have a complete ear examination including an audiogram and be referred to an otolaryngologist. The ear canal can be abnormally narrow (stenotic) throughout its entire length or narrowed for only a short segment. Segmental stenosis usually occurs at the bony-cartilaginous junction and may be mild or severe enough to appear as only a dimple within the meatus. The tympanic membrane and middle ear beyond the stenosis may be normal or deformed.

The narrowed ear canal should be kept free of wax and debris to prevent occlusion, which will result in a conductive hearing loss. Mineral oil, antibiotic drops, or peroxide applied weekly will keep the wax soft and permit easy cleaning of the canal with a curette or Water-Pik®. If the canal can be kept open and free of infection, no further treatment is required. Canal stenosis associated with persistent hearing loss or recurrent infection requires a referral to an otolaryngologist for surgical correction to widen the external ear canal.

Complete failure of canal formulation, or atresia, causes a 50-60 dB conductive hearing loss by blocking the transmission of sound to the inner ear. The area in which the tympanic membrane should be located behind the canal atresia usually consists of a bony plate attached to the underlying ossicles. Any child with canal atresia should have an audiogram. If the deformity is unilateral and hearing is normal in the other ear, no further treatment is required. With preferential seating in school and some special attention, the child with unilateral microtia and one normal ear will have normal speech, social, and intellectual development.

Since the child with bilateral atresia will have at least a 50-60 dB hearing deficit in both ears, intervention is required for normal speech development. Hearing aids should be placed early (less than six months of age) and their use continued until surgical correction is considered, usually around five years of age. Since the facial nerve and middle ear structure may also be abnormal in the child with atresia, the surgical repair carries some risk of damaging these structures. For this reason, repair of unilateral atresia is almost never considered, and only one ear is repaired in the child with a bilateral deformity. The decision to operate on the second ear, after successful repair of the first side, is best delayed until the patient is an adult and he can participate in the decision.

First branchial cleft anomalies may present with intermittent drainage from the ear canal and a cystic mass or cutaneous sinus at the angle of the mandible or behind the pinna. These patients should be referred to an otolaryngologist for treatment of these malformations whose tracts often course near, or even between, the branches of the facial nerve. Incomplete excision of the skin-lined sac and tract will only result in recurrence of the lesion and repeated infections.

Middle Ear

Middle ear anomalies may be associated with (and, in fact, heralded by) external ear anomalies but also may be found as isolated entities. Patients with craniofacial anomalies such as Treacher-Collins, Goldenhar's, and Crouzon's or Apert's syndrome frequently have ossicular anomalies. Often the appearance of the tympanic membrane is perfectly normal, but there is almost always a conductive hearing loss. Ossicular anomalies may vary from mildly deformed ossicles that function well to a total absence of part or all of the ossicles. The bones may be partially or totally fused, causing immobility and hearing loss. Ossicular anomalies are frequently associated with an aberrant course of the facial nerve in the temporal bone. However, this anomaly is usually not associated with any abnormal facial nerve function. The absence of the oval or round window is rarely seen.

If the hearing loss caused by a middle ear anomaly, either unilateral or bilateral, is sufficient to interfere with the child's social or intellectual function, the patient should be referred to an otolaryngologist for consideration of hearing aid placement or surgical correction. All middle ear anomalies causing a conductive hearing loss are potentially correctable. The amount of hearing improvement depends on the severity of the malformation, often determined only during exploration of the middle ear.

A middle ear anomaly not associated with hearing loss, but that can be a nuisance and lead to a potential disaster, is the presence of a high jugular bulb in the posterior-inferior portion of the middle ear. The high jugular bulb usually has no bony coverage, so it appears as a smooth dark blue mass behind the tympanic membrane. This anomaly causes no problems unless it is disturbed during instrumentation of the tympanic membrane or middle ear. If a patient with a high jugular bulb requires a tympanocentesis, it should be performed by an otolaryngologist who can treat the ear adequately if the bulb is entered. External canal packing and, rarely, middle ear exploration are required for proper treatment of a punctured jugular bulb. If massive bleeding is encountered after a myringotomy in the primary care physician's office, the ear canal should be packing firmly with Vaseline® gauze and the patient referred immediately to an otolaryngologist.

Inner Ear

Inner ear anomalies are less common than anomalies of the external or middle ear. The vast majority of patients with congenital sensorineural hearing loss have no visible anomaly of the external, middle or inner ear. Some of these patients, however, have associated disorders in other organ systems. For this reason, any child with a congenital sensorineural hearing loss should have a complete ear examination and special attention given to the renal, cardiovascular, and endocrine systems as well. The inner ear anomalies cause a sensorineural hearing loss that is most often stable, but occasionally the hearing loss will be found to fluctuate.

The inner ear deformities range from minor anomalies of the membranous labyrinth to total absence of the bony cochlear and vestibular labyrinth. Congenital anomalies of the spiral ganglion, eighth nerve, and central auditory pathways also occur. Conventional audiometry and brainstem-evoked responses can be used to determine the hearing level and, in some cases, the site of the anomaly. Computed tomography of the temporal bone can define the bony details of the inner ear malformation but does not give information regarding the structure or function of the membranous labyrinth. Treatment of inner ear anomalies generally involves correction of any underlying metabolic or inflammatory condition and amplification with a hearing aid.

Congenital Deafness

Congenital deafness occurs in approximately one of 1,500 to one of 2,000 live births. The frequency is likely to increase, as our knowledge of neonatal diseases and their management increases and survival of premature infants improves. Hereditary congenital deafness may be transmitted as a dominant or recessive trait. Recessive transmission accounts for 90% of genetic congenital deafness. Other causes include factors that affect the ear during pregnancy or shortly after birth such as *rubella virus, cytomegalovirus, birth anoxia, hyperbiliruninemia*, and exposure to ototoxic or recreational drugs.

Congenital deafness may occur in association with integumentary diseases and anomalies. The best known of these disorders is *Waardenberg's syndrome*, which accounts for 2% of congenital deafness. Patients with complete expression of the syndrome have a white forelock, pseudohypertelorism, and confluent eyebrows. Some of these patients also have patchy areas of vitiligo. Approximately 20% of patients with Waardenberg's syndrome have a sensorineural hearing loss that tends to stabilize over time. Vestibular involvement is poorly defined. Another sensorineural hearing loss syndrome involving the integument is albinism. These patients also display nystagmus and have photophobia. In *Leopard's syndrome*, areas of cutaneous hyperpigmentation are present in addition to a sensorineural loss. Freckles are present all over the body but spare mucosal surfaces. One-half of affected males have hypospadias and pulmonary artery stenosis. Growth retardation may be present as well. Other integumentary characteristics such as baldness, hyperkeratosis, and fingernail abnormalities have been reported in sporadic cases of hearing impairment.

Hearing deficits may be associated with ophthalmologic problems. The most commonly identified disorder of this group is *Usher's syndrome*. These patients have a moderate to severe sensorineural hearing loss, vestibular disturbances, and progressive retinitis pigmentosa. Vision deteriorates progressively over several decades, but the hearing loss usually remains stable. Retinal degeneration, retinal detachment, and myopia have also been reported occasionally in association with a sensorineural hearing deficit.

Endocrine and metabolic disorders have also been associated with sensorineural hearing loss. In *Pendred's syndrome*, patients have a goiter that usually appears before puberty, as well as a sensorineural hearing loss. Thyroid function is normal in most cases, but hypothyroidism may be present. The severity of the hearing deficit varies and may be progressive. Patients with mucopolysaccharidoses such as *Hunter's* or *Hurler's syndrome* often have sensorineural losses, but frequently there is a conductive or mixed (sensorineural-conductive) loss. These patients have a very high incidence of secretory otitis media secondary to cranial-skeletal deformity and intracellular deposits of acid mucopolysaccharides in nasopharyngeal tissue. The conductive loss may be progressive as deposits build up on the ossicular chain. Lipodystrophy (*Tay Sachs*) and defects in copper metabolism (*Wilson's disease*) may also cause sensorineural hearing loss.

Renal insufficiency and sensorineural hearing loss, both of which are progressive, are present in *Alport's disease*. This syndrome accounts for 1% of all genetic deafness. The hearing loss affects the middle and high frequencies and usually appears between the age of 10 and 20 years. Urine analysis shows variable degrees of hematuria, pyuria, and proteinuria. *Renal tubular acidosis* is also associated with a progressive sensorineural hearing loss. In these patients, the use of ototoxic drugs should be restricted to life-threatening situations, since the renal failure may cause these agents to reach higher blood levels, resulting in additional sensorineural hearing impairment.

There is no medical or surgical treatment for the vast majority of cases of congenital sensorineural hearing loss. The child should be treated with hearing aid amplification as soon as the loss is detected and characterized. The rare case of fluctuating sensorineural hearing loss related to a congenital cochlear defect may respond to middle ear and mastoid exploration and decompression of inner ear fluid.

DEGENERATIVE DISORDERS

Otosclerosis is a degenerative disease that causes a progressive conductive hearing loss, but it may have an associated sensorineural component as well. Otosclerosis is a familial disorder that occurs most commonly in young Caucasian adults and rarely in childhood. In the otosclerotic ear, an abnormal growth of bone is responsible for fixation of the stapes footplate to the oval window, eliminating the mechanical advantage of the ossicular chain. The sensorineural component is usually found when the bony capsule of the labyrinth is involved with the otosclerotic process. The reason for the sensorineural impairment in these patients is unclear. Metabolic toxins in the cochlea from an adjacent otosclerotic focus is one possible etiology for the sensorineural component. When otosclerosis is present in a child, it is often associated with bony disorder *osteogenesis imperfecta*. These patients have fragile bones, blue sclerae, and a conductive hearing loss that may be unilateral or bilateral. Children with otosclerosis should be referred to an otolaryngologist for possible correction of the conductive hearing impairment by stapedectomy.

SECRETORY OTITIS MEDIA (OTITIS MEDIA WITH EFFUSION)

Secretory otitis media, serous otitis media, and otitis media with effusion are all terms for one of the most frequently encountered conditions seen in the primary care physician's office. Secretory otitis media is the accumulation of serous or mucous fluid within the middle ear space. It may occur concurrently with an upper respiratory infection, after treatment of acute otitis media, associated with a nasopharyngeal neoplasm, or without a known cause. Chronic secretory otitis media is the most common otologic condition seen during childhood. Children under six years of age have the greatest incidence, and the rate of occurrence decreases with age. It is an uncommon condition in young adults and is usually only present following barotrauma from scuba diving or flying during an upper respiratory infection. Because secretory otitis media is painless, causes a mild to moderate hearing loss, and is often only associated with vague symptoms, it can go undetected for months or years. The actual incidence of secretory otitis media is therefore probably far greater than is currently appreciated by statistics derived from cases seen in physician's offices.

TABLE 1-2 Causes of Secretory Otitis Media

Inflammation
 Infection
  Viral infection (upper respiratory infection)
  Bacterial infections (nasopharyngitis)
  Fungal, etc.
 Allergy
 Pollutants
  Smoke
  Dust
  Fumes from crafts
 Low humidity (dry respiratory mucosa)
Obstruction
 Adenoid hypertrophy
Tumors
 Benign
 Malignant
Anatomic deformities
 Cleft palate
 Craniofacial anomalies (Crouzon's)
 Down's syndrome
Systemic diseases and endocrine disorders
 Glycogen storage
 Mucopolysaccharoidosis
 Amyloidosis
 Sarcoidosis
 Heart failure
 Renal failure
 Pregnancy
 Hypothyroidism
Trauma
 Surgery
  Nasal
  Nasopharyngeal
 Pharyngeal burns
  Heat
  Caustic
 Tubes
  Nasogastric tubes
  Nasotracheal tubes
 Blunt and sharp trauma to nasopharynx
 Barotrauma
  Airplane
  Scuba diving

Etiology

While secretory otitis media has been attributed to a myriad of etiologies (Table 1-2), the pathogenesis of the effusion is the same in most instances. Secretory otitis media develops when the mucociliary transport system is significantly altered or when the outflow tract for secretions is obstructed. The mucociliary transport system may be disturbed in several ways. The quality or quantity of the secretions may change as in allergy or in upper respiratory infection states. Ciliary function (*Kartagener's syndrome*) may be inadequate to clear the fluid. The outflow tract may be affected by obstruction of the eustachian tube (by adenoid tissue or nasopharyngeal tumors) or by physiologic dysfunction caused by alteration of the presurre dynamics in the nasopharynx.

Several clinical conditions predispose children and adolescents to secretory otitis media. The most common is the actual configuration of the cranial base and the anatomy of the eustachian tube in the young person. The horizontal position of the tube in the child is not optimal for middle ear drainage and permits nasopharyngeal reflux. In addition, the muscular function of the tensor veli palatini may not be maximal. The cartilage of the child's auditory tube is more flaccid than in the adult, offering less support to the tube and making it more susceptible to nasopharyngeal pressure fluctuations. As the child grows, the position of the eustachian tube becomes more vertical and cartilage support becomes firm, making eustachian tube function more efficient.

Craniofacial deformities (the most common of which is cleft palate) also predispose young children and adolescents to secretory otitis media. Nearly all patients with unrepaired cleft palates (submucous, partial, or complete) have secretory otitis media; many cases of secretory otitis media persist, even after the palate has been repaired. In a cleft palate deformity, the tensor palatini muscle does not have a normal midline attachment and functions poorly in opening the eustachian tube. Any craniofacial deformity in which the maxilla is short or narrow is also associated with a high incidence of secretory otitis media. This is most likely related to the anatomic configuration of the palate and nasopharynx, resulting in poor function of the eustachian tube.

Any *inflammatory process* in the upper respiratory tract predisposes patients to secretory otitis media. Acute secretory otitis media is most commonly seen during a viral upper respiratory infection. The condition usually resolves spontaneously as the signs and symptoms of the upper respiratory infection subside. Secretory otitis media is also encountered in association with localized or diffuse bacterial infection of the upper respiratory tract. Patients with sinusitis, pharyngitis, or bronchitis commonly have secretory otitis media. While the actual bacterial infection may be confined primarily to one area, inflammation is usually present throughout the entire respiratory tract, including the eustachian tube and middle ear mucosa. Rarely, secretory otitis media is associated with a fungal or parasitic infection of the upper respiratory tract. As the primary infection resolves with appropriate therapy, the middle ear effusion usually clears, although it may persist to become chronic.

Allergic inflammation in the respiratory tract is also a frequent cause of secretory otitis media in patients with an atopic disorder. The secretory otitis media may be either seasonal, fluctuating with the severity of the allergic symptoms, or perennial, depending on the allergic diathesis.

Inhalation of *irritating substances* can cause diffuse inflammation throughout the upper respiratory tract and contribute to the development of secretory otitis media. Inflammation affects the mucociliary transport system by increasing the volume of secretions as well as by altering the viscosity and elasticity of the mucus. *Smoke* from cigarettes, fireplaces, and, increasingly in young people, marihuana causes varying degrees of respiratory tract inflammation. Since marihuana smoke is rarely filtered, it may enter the nasopharynx at high temperatures and cause a first-degree pharyngeal burn as well. Rebreathing the exhaled smoke exacerbates the problem. Certain volatile household and hobby fumes may also be very irritating to the nasopharyngeal mucosa when inhaled.

Systemic diseases that affect tissue composition or retention of fluids also predispose young people to middle ear effusions. Secretory otitis media may be found in the middle ear of patients with hypothyroidism, amyloidosis, renal failure, heart failure, mucopolysaccharidosis, or sarcoidosis, and during pregnancy. In *Kartagener's syndrome* and similar conditions in which ciliary motility is impaired, middle ear secretions are not cleared from the middle ear cleft, and secretory otitis media results.

Nasopharyngeal masses may alter eustachian tube function by blocking the tube orifice or by altering the pressure-equalizing function of the nasopharyngeal-eustachian tube complex. The most frequently encountered nasopharyngeal mass affecting eustachian tube function is adenoid tissue. Adenoid hypertrophy may result from repeated infections or in upper respiratory allergic states.

A less common, but still important, cause of nasopharyngeal obstruction is the presence of both benign and malignant tumors. Benign tumors such as nasopharyngeal and angiofibromas, antralchoanal polyps, and minor salivary gland tumors may cause secretory otitis media. The most common malignant tumors found in the nasopharynx include rhabdomyosarcoma and lymphoma; rarely, nasopharyngeal carcinoma is found. Secretory otitis media caused by a tumor is usually unilateral in the early phases while the tumor is small but become bilateral as the tumor grows.

Trauma to the nasopharynx may injure the eustachian tube directly or indirectly (by locally spreading inflammation and edema). Secretory otitis media is common in patients with indwelling nasotracheal or nasogastric tubes and may appear after only two or three days of tube placement. Temporal bone fractures or surgical trauma in the region of the eustachian tube as a result of cleft palate repair or construction of a pharyngeal flap for velopharyngeal incompetence can also cause secretory otitis media.

The role of *microorganisms* (both viral and bacterial) in the development of secretory otitis media is controversial. While secretory otitis media has not been traditionally considered an infectious disease, several investigators have found pathogenic bacteria or viruses in a significant percentage of patients with middle ear effusion. Whether these organisms represent a primary infection or the residual of an incompletely treated acute otitis media is unclear.

Diagnosis

A comprehensive approach to the management of secretory otitis media requires recognition of the middle ear effusion, as well as a complete search for an underlying predisposing condition. A high level of suspicion is important when examining children at risk for secretory otitis media, because it is usually painless and is only associated with vague complaints. Secretory otitis media should be suspected in any child who appears inattentive, does not follow directions, or daydreams in school. A child who says "what?" constantly or who adjusts the television to uncomfortable levels for others in the room may have secretory otitis media. In very young children, parents are the most reliable observers and are usually the first to suspect a mild hearing loss by noticing inappropriate or absent responses to sounds as well as "clumsy" movements.

Secretory otitis media is most effectively diagnosed by pneumatic otoscopy. Too often, the focus of attention in otoscopic evaluation is the tympanic membrane itself. However, through the translucent membrane, fluid may be seen in the middle ear space. The effusion may be amber, blue, or brown. The presence of air in the middle ear space will be exhibited by bubbles and air-fluid levels. However, if the fluid is clear and completely fills the middle ear space, it is difficult to visualize. Pneumatic otoscopy may be the only means of detecting clear fluid through the demonstration of the decreased mobility of the tympanic membrane. Fluid in the middle ear is always associated with negative pressure in the middle ear space from absorption of oxygen. The result is retraction of the tympanic membrane, which leads to two subtle signs of secretory otitis media: the short process of the malleus becomes more prominent and the long process appears foreshortened.

Tympanometry has become a useful tool in the management of secretory otitis media. If there is no change in acoustic impedance of an ear over the range of -400 to +400 mm H_2O, there is an 80 to 90% probability of secretory otitis media. If the point of maximum compliance is in the negative range, the probability drops to approximately 50%.

Complications

Secretory otitis media is an important problem in children and young adults because of its common occurrence and potential for long-term problems. Although its early effects may be mild and subtle, secretory otitis media may lead to serious complications that can be difficult or impossible to remedy.

Fluid in the middle ear changes the mechanical properties of the tympanic membrane and ossicular complex, causing a conductive hearing loss that may range from 5 dB (mild) to 40 dB (moderate). The loss may be stable or may fluctuate as the fluid varies in amount and consistency.

Hearing losses attributable to secretory otitis media may be responsible for delayed language and speech development. Affected children may begin talking later than their peers, have poor articulation, and demonstrate slow vocabulary development. These children also score poorly on tests that require reception and processing of auditory stimuli and may have difficulty producing verbal responses. Since our educational system is so heavily dependent on verbal language skills, secretory otitis media creates a serious educational disadvantage for any child. It is also possible that critical periods of auditory development may pass during corresponding periods of auditory deprivation from secretory otitis media. If this occurs, auditory learning may be affected throughout an entire lifetime.

Mild hearing loss may also be associated with noticeable behavioral problems. Young children with secretory otitis media may wake frequently at night and be irritable throughout the day. Preschool- and school-age children alike may exhibit dramatic swings of behavior, ranging from hyperactivity to withdrawal whenever fluid is present. Older children often seen to be impatient and "not themselves."

Coordination may also be affected by fluid in the middle ear. A child with secretory otitis media is often described as clumsy or as "falling a lot." This may account for the impression that children with secretory otitis media appear to begin walking later than their normal peers. The balance problem may be a sign that brings about a visit to the primary care physician and the discovery of secretory otitis media. Caution should be taken in the interpretation of symptoms of clumsiness in a child with secretory otitis media, since these symptoms may signal another more serious neurological problem.

Secretory otitis media provides an excellent culture medium for bacteria in the middle ear and is often associated with recurrent bouts of acute otitis media. The middle ear effusion may be colonized directly from the nasopharynx or via bloodstream from another distant source.

Secretory otitis media always causes retraction of the tympanic membrane. Initially this may be only a mild retraction with minimal inward rotation of the malleus. As retraction progresses, the tympanic membrane may begin to adhere to the promontory and the long process of the incus. Deeper retraction causes ossicular erosion and formation of a retraction pocket. Ossicular erosion is associated with a 40 to 60 dB (moderate to severe) conductive hearing loss that may require major reconstructive surgery for correction. The formation of a retraction pocket in the tympanic membrane may lead to the development of a cholesteatoma (skin-lined sac) that expands and destroys the structures of the middle ear and mastoid.

The complications of secretory otitis media, ranging from mild to severe, can be prevented by having a high index of suspicion when examining children at risk of having secretory otitis media, making an earlier diagnosis of the process, and treating both the secretory otitis media and any predisposing causes.

Treatment

The medical therapy of secretory otitis media is directed toward the treatment of any underlying predisposing condition. Since inflammation is the most common condition leading to the development of secretory otitis media, medication are directed at the source of the inflammation. Antibiotic therapy may help determine any bacterial inflammation in the nasopharynx and the middle ear cleft. Antihistamines and decongestants have been used extensively in children with secretory otitis media, but have no proven efficacy; their observed, but not proven, benefit may be a result of viscosity changes that facilitate clearance of the mucus. Any benefit of their use needs to weighed against the side effects that include mood and behavior changes, especially in young children. Short courses of systemic corticosteroids and local steroids nasal sprays have their advocates, but long-term benefits remain questionable. If secretory otitis media is associated with recurrent acute otitis media, bacterial suppression with a broad-spectrum antibiotic, such as sulfamethoxazole, 500 mg twice a day, or amoxicillin, 250 mg once or twice daily for six weeks, may permit clearing of the middle ear. Regardless of the medication given, the actual effective medical therapy in many of these patients may be "tincture of time."

If a middle ear effusion remains without noticeable improvement after six weeks of medical therapy, consideration should be given for referral to an otolaryngologist. This six-week time frame is not a fixed rule. The referral of each child should be individualized and based on the condition of the middle ear, the presence of any complications, and the degree of developmental or educational impairment. If the effusion is chronic and appropriate medical therapy has failed to clear an effusion over a three month period, a myringotomy and placement of a ventilation tube are usually recommended. An incision is made in the tympanic membrane, the middle ear fluid aspirated and a tube is placed in the incision. The purpose of the hollow tube is to keep the incision in the tympanic membrane open to permit equalization of middle ear pressure and to prevent reaccumulation of fluid. If the mucociliary transport system and eustachian tube have returned to normal function by the time the tubes extrude spontaneously (usually in 6 to 12 months), the middle ear will remain free of fluid after the incision in the tympanic membrane heals. In several studies, adenoidectomy has been shown to be an effective adjuvant in children requiring multiple sets of tubes for recurrent serous otitis media.

ACUTE OTITIS MEDIA

Etiology

Acute suppurative otitis media is one of the most commonly seen acute infectious conditions in the primary care practice, second only to upper respiratory tract infection. It is caused by bacterial infection in the middle ear space. Acute otitis media may occur as an isolated process but most often presents a few days after the onset of an upper respiratory tract infection. Patients with chronic secretory otitis media or with immune deficiencies are also subject to repeated bouts of the acute condition.

The organism that most commonly causes acute otitis media in any age child is *Streptococcus pneumoniae*. In children under five years of age, non-typeable *Hemophilus influenzae* is seen in a significant percentage of patients. Less frequently, group A ß-hemolytic streptococcus, *Staphylococcus aureus* and gram-negative enteric organisms are causative agents. The *enteric organisms* are most common in patients with altered or decreased defenses (such as neonates) and in children with immune-deficiency states, aplastic anemia, or malignancies requiring chemotherapy. Rarely, *tuberculosis* or *fungi* may infect the middle ear. *Viruses* have been cultured and implicated as etiologic agents in some series of children with acute otitis media.

Diagnosis

Acute otitis media should be suspected in any child with deep acute ear pain, irritability, or lethargy. The severe pain of acute otitis media develops rapidly and is usually accompanied by fever and loss of hearing. In some children, the pain is not severe or the level of pain intolerance may be high; in these cases the first sign of the infection may be sudden ear discharge from a spontaneous perforation of the tympanic membrane. Lethargy may be the only sign of infection in the neonate. Fever may be absent, even in the most severe infections.

Acute otitis media is best diagnosed by otoscopy. Pulling on the pinna to introduce the otoscope speculum does not increase the discomfort, as it does in external otitis. In the early stages of acute otitis media, the tympanic membrane may be only slightly hyperemic with normal contours. However, tympanic membrane mobility is almost always decreased in these patients. As the infection progresses, the tympanic membrane thickens, becomes more inflamed, and bulges laterally on either side of the malleus. Later, the landmarks of the tympanic membrane become totally unrecognizable as the drum bulges laterally to leave the umbo "buried" deep to the surface of the tympanic membrane.

Occasionally, blebs or blisters filled with a clear fluid appear on the lateral surface of the tympanic membrane. Originally, the occurrence of bullous myringitis was attributed to a *Mycoplasma* infection. Recent evidence has shown that this entity is really a form of acute otitis media and is caused by the same organisms responsible for the conventionally appearing acute otitis media.

Complications

During the acute phase of *acute otitis media,* purulent exudate in the middle ear space causes a conductive hearing loss. The hearing loss usually resolves completely as the infection subsides. However, the inflammatory process may stimulate fibrosis, hyalinization, and calcium deposition in mucoid material that can adhere to any of the bony surfaces of the middle ear as well as the medial aspect of the tympanic membrane. These *tympanosclerotic plaques,* when they are on the tympanic membrane, appear as irregular patches of white material that are often incorrectly called "scars." Tympanosclerosis is not usually associated with a measurable hearing deficit. Rarely, large plaques can impede tympanic membrane mobility or fix the ossicular chain, causing a conductive hearing impairment.

In some cases of acute otitis media, the tympanic membrane may perforate spontaneously as a result of tissue necrosis during the acute phase of the infection. These *perforations* are usually small, occur in the central portion of the pars tensa, and heal spontaneously as the infection resolves. Large perforations, however, often do not heal. The ossicular chain may also be affected by the inflammatory process. Necrosis of the long process of the incus is the most common ossicular sequela of acute otitis media. Both persistent perforation of the tympanic membrane and ossicular necrosis or discontinuity are accompanied by a conductive hearing loss. *Tuberculosis* otitis media usually causes multiple small persistent perforations.

As a tympanic membrane perforation heals, squamous epithelium may grow into the middle ear, forming a skin-lined sac, or *cholesteatoma* that collects desquamated epithelial debris. These cystic masses, which continue to expand, can destroy the surrounding structures in the middle ear, mastoid, and inner ear (see the following section on chronic otitis media).

Facial nerve paralysis may occur suddenly during acute otitis media. Since one half of all children have an incomplete bony covering over a portion of the facial nerve in the middle ear, this exposed portion of the nerve is vulnerable to inflammation and injury during acute otitis media. When first observed, the facial nerve paralysis may be partial or complete and usually involves all three divisions on the infected side. Facial nerve function usually recovers completely with proper management, consisting of an immediate wide myringotomy (for drainage and culture) and intravenous antibiotic therapy.

A sterile inflammatory process may occur in the adjacent inner ear in acute otitis media. This *serous labyrinthitis* is usually associated with mild vertigo, but hearing is unaffected. However, if bacteria invade the inner ear through the oval or round windows, acute suppurative labyrinthitis develops. This process results in severe vertigo and profound sensorineural hearing loss and may spread intracranially, resulting in meningitis.

In all cases of acute otitis media, the mastoid air cells are affected by the inflammatory process and are filled with purulent exudate similar to that seen in the middle ear. However, acute coalescent mastoiditis (*acute mastoid osteomyelitis*) may develop as a complication of acute otitis media. When this occurs, the septae of the mastoid air-cell system necrose and the air-cell system fills with granulation tissue that may break through the overlying mastoid cortex. This condition is associated with severe pain behind the ear, swelling and redness over the mastoid region, and inferolateral displacement of the auricle (Fig. 1-11). On otoscopic examination, the posterior-superior wall of the external canal appears to sag forward. While mastoid radiographs of all children with acute otitis media will show opacification of the mastoid air cells, the bony space will be absent in cases of coalescent mastoiditis. In rare cases, the mastoid tip necroses, and purulent material dissects into the planes of the neck, causing a bulge anterior to the sternocleidomastoid muscle (*Bezold's abscess*). The infection may also reach the air cells of the medial portion of the temporal bone by necrosis of the perilabyrinthine air cells, causing *petrosal apicitis*. In this condition, also known as *Gradenigo's syndrome*, there is pain in the distribution of the trigeminal nerve and paralysis of the abducens nerve. Both acute coalescent mastoiditis and petrositis require intravenous antibiotics and prompt surgical drainage of the infection.

The most common intracranial complication of acute otitis media is *meningitis*. It most often occurs when the diagnosis and treatment of acute otitis media is delayed. It may also occur even though appropriate doses of an oral antibiotic are instituted for acute otitis media. Otitis meningitis can be accompanied by any of the typical neurologic complications that occur with meningitis from any source: brain damage, abscess formation, and cranial nerve dysfunction. Sensorineural deafness develops in approximately 7% of patients with *H. influenzae* meningitis. Other intracranial complications that may occur with acute otitis media include cerebritis, epidural abscess, brain abscess, and lateral sinus thrombosis. Otitis hydrocephalus occurs as a complication of thrombophlebitis of the petrosal sinus. CT scans are very useful in the early detection of intracranial complications and should be performed in any child with acute otitis media complaining of a localized headache or displaying a change in mental

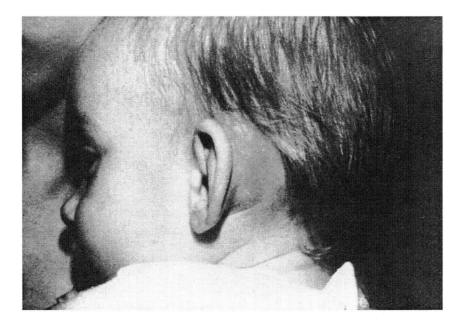

Figure 1–11. Child with coalescent mastoiditis. Note the downward and lateral displacement of the auricle. (From Potsic WP, Handler SD, Wetmore RF: Ear, Nose, Throat and Mouth. In: Rudolph A (ed). Pediatrics. 19th ed. Norwalk, CT, Appleton & Lange, 1991.)

status or signs of a focal neurologic deficit. Treatment of any of these complications requires intravenous antibiotics, wide myringotomy, and drainage of any intracranial abscess.

Treatment

Treatment of acute otitis media consists of 10 days of an antibiotic that is likely to be effective against the common organisms for that age group. Since *S. pneumonia* and *H. influenzae* are the most common causes of acute otitis media in children, either ampicillin or amoxicillin is the drug of choice. In older children, penicillin is usually effective. However, since *H. influenzae* may be more common in older children than previously thought, ampicillin (or amoxicillin) should probably be the drug of choice in this group, too. Relief of pain, fever, and malaise usually occurs six to eight hours. after treatment has been instituted. Recently ampicillin-resistant *H. influenzae* has begun to account for as much as 30% of the *H. influenzae* acute otitis media reported in some areas. If a child with acute otitis media is not responding to appropriate antibiotic therapy as expected, switching to an agent that is not affected by the ß-lactamase produced by the *H. influenzae* (such as sulfamethoxazole and erythromycin, trimethoprim and sulfa, amoxicillin and clavuline acid, or cefaclor) may be indicated. Antibiotic therapy should be given for 10 days; the ear should be monitored until all signs of infection and middle ear fluid have disappeared.

Antihistamine-decongestant preparations, and nasal decongestant sprays are of no proven benefit in the treatment of acute otitis media. The application of heat and anesthetic eardrops to the ear may be soothing but are of no therapeutic value.

Tympanocentesis may be helpful in managing the child with acute otitis media who is not responding to conventional antibiotic therapy. This approach is especially important for any patient, such as a newborn infant or immunosuppressed child, suspected of harboring a resistant or unusual organism. The ear canal is sterilized with an iodine-containing solution or alcohol. A 22-gauge spinal needle is introduced through one of the inferior quadrants of the tympanic membrane into the middle ear, and the fluid is aspirated into a syringe (Fig. 1-12). Immediate Gram stain and later culture and sensitivity results will indicate selection of specific antibiotics. Myringotomy for pain relief alone is of limited value and does not appear to hasten the resolution of acute otitis media.

Apparent or impending intracranial complications concomitant with acute otitis media warrant referral of the patient to an otolaryngologist. Such cases require immediate surgical intervention, the least of which would be a wide inferior myringotomy.

Children with three episodes of acute otitis media that recur quickly are candidates for antibiotic prophylaxis with either sulfamethoxazole or amoxicillin in a daily dose approximately one-half the therapeutic dose. Other antibiotics may also be tried for prophylaxis. Vaccines against common pathogens have no proven efficacy in the management of recurrent acute otitis media. A referral to an otolaryngologist should be considered for breakthrough infection, intolerance to antibiotic medication, or prolonged problems with recurrent acute otitis media. Surgical management including placement of ventilation tubes may be indicated in these patients. Ventilation tubes do not prevent upper respiratory infection, however, they do prevent the accumulation of fluid during thoseinfections that frequently lead to acute otitis media.

Drainage from an ear with a ventilation tube in place may be the result of exposure of the ear to contaminated water (i.e., swimming pool)

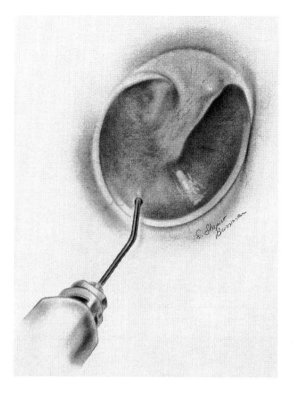

Figure 1–12. Tympanocentesis is performed with a syringe and a 22-guage spinal needle inserted through the inferior portion of the tympanic membrane.

or may be associated with a bacterial upper respiratory infection. Treatment should include the use of antibiotic ear drops several times daily and a broad spectrum oral antibiotic.

CHRONIC OTITIS MEDIA

Etiology

Chronic otitis media is defined as a long-standing (greater than six weeks) perforation of the tympanic membrane or the presence of cholesteatoma. The perforation may have occurred spontaneously (in rare cases) or as a result of infection or trauma. In children with chronic perforations, the middle ear space may be free of infection and the ear termed "dry." Or, there may be an infection of the middle ear mucosa with otorrhea and the ear called "wet" or "moist." Infections of the middle ear are usually caused by *Pseudomonas* and *Staphylococcus aureus*. The infection presents with a foul, profuse, and mucopurulent otorrhea. Pain and fever are usually absent because the purulent material is draining through the perforation.

A cholesteatoma is a skin-lined sac that collects desquamated squamous debris. A cholesteatoma may occur in association with a perforated tympanic membrane in the acquired condition, or it may be present behind an intact membrane in the congenital condition. The sacs most commonly develop from the inward migration of epithelium at the edge of a perforation. On rare occasions, a cholesteatoma may have no connection to a tympanic membrane perforation; these are thought to be squamous epithelial rests trapped behind the tympanic membrane during embryologic development, termed *congenital cholesteatomas*. Often a chronic low-grade infection within the cyst contributes to the accumulated debris. As the debris builds up and the cholesteatoma expands, the mass may destroy the structures of the middle ear and extend to the mastoid air-cell system. Cholesteatomas may extend along the floor of the middle cranial fossa, under the temporal lobe, and along the perilabyrinthine air cells to the apex of the temporal bone. Destruction of the bones of the middle ear and mastoid is most likely aided by osteolytic enzymes released by the cellular degradation and bacteria in the cholesteatoma.

Diagnosis

The diagnosis of chronic otitis media is made by the otoscopic evaluation. The tympanic membrane perforation, cholesteatoma debris, or both are usually easily seen. If otorrhea is present, the purulent material may need to be cleaned from the external canal with a suction or cotton-tip applicator before the pathology can be visualized. Particular care should be taken to visualize the pars flaccida, where a small perforation or cholesteatoma may be difficult to see. The squamous debris of a cholesteatoma appears as flaky white material at the edge of the perforation or as a smooth white mass behind a translucent tympanic membrane. The limits of the cholesteatoma in the mastoid are best defined by CT.

Complications

The recurrent and persistent ear infections commonly associated with chronic otitis media can lead to all the complications seen in patients with acute otitis media. The management of these complications is the same as for those secondary to the acute condition, with the additional problem of treating the tympanic membrane perforation or cholesteatoma.

Treatment

Chronic otitis media with infection in the middle ear is most effectively treated with eardrops containing antibiotics effective against *Pseudomonas* and *Staphylococcus*, which are most commonly found in these patients. Eardrops containing acetic acid are also effective therapy but are painful to the ear, making patient compliance low in children. Proper cleansing of the ear prior to instillation of the drops will hasten resolution of the infection. Any otorrhea in the meatus should be suctioned out or absorbed with a cotton-tip applicator. The drops can then be placed in an open meatus to flow down the ear canal, straightened by pulling the auricle posteriorly and superiorly. Systemic antibiotics have a limited role in the treatment of chronic otitis media. They are best reserved for cases in which local therapy has failed to clear up the infection or in which the process has spread to surrounding tissues, causing local cellulitis or adenitis. All children with chronic otitis media should be referred to an otolaryngologist after a 10-day course of medical therapy or sooner if a complication such as facial nerve paralysis or vertigo occurs.

Medical treatment of chronic otitis media eliminates the active infection but does not alter the basic pathologic condition of the ear — perforation of the drum or the presence of cholesteatoma. Treatment of the perforated tympanic membrane requires surgical reconstruction of the tympanic membrane and ossicular chain (tympanoplasty). Cholesteatomas must be either completely excised or exteriorized to prevent continued expansion and progressive destruction of the middle ear structures and temporal bone. This approach often requires surgical exposure of the mastoid (mastoidectomy). After complete excision of a cholesteatoma is accomplished, surgical reconstruction of the mastoid, ossicles, and tympanic membrane (tympanomastoidoplasty) may be possible to restore the anatomic and functional integrity of the ear.

EXTERNAL OTITIS

External otitis, or otitis externa, is a condition involving an active inflammation of the outer ear and ear canal. While this problem is most often only a mild nuisance, occasional cases are serious and potentially dangerous.

Etiology

Moisture in the ear canal leading to maceration of the skin lining, making it susceptible to infection, is the most common cause of external otitis. Frequent swimming, hairwashing, and even long exposure to a humid environment may provide sufficient moisture to the ear canal to predispose it to develop external otitis. Children with less or drier wax than normal, either naturally or as a result of a regional radiation therapy, appear to have a higher incidence of external otitis. This correlation leads us to suspect that a normal amount and consistency of cerumen may be a significant factor in preventing external otitis.

Local trauma to the ear canal is a common cause of external otitis. A fingernail, cotton-tip applicator, paper clip, or foreign body may lacerate the ear canal and permit infection to take hold once the skin barrier has been violated. Large foreign bodies may prevent the exit of cerumen and desquamated debris from the ear canal. This retained debris will contribute to the occurrence of external otitis. A large plug of impacted cerumen may cause external otitis in the same manner.

Occasionally, purulent secretions of acute otitis media will contribute to the occurrence of external otitis. A large plug of impacted cerumen may cause external otitis in the same manner.

Occasionally, purulent secretions of acute otitis media will drain through a spontaneous perforation of the tympanic membrane. These secretions may irritate the external canal, causing external otitis as a complication of the original condition.

The condition of the skin in the ear canal may be altered by local or generalized *dermatologic* disorders. Psoriasis, seborrhea, eczema, and contact dermatitis (from hairsprays or other chemicals) may predispose the patient to infection in the ear canal.

External otitis is most frequently caused by *Pseudomonas aeruginosa* and *Staphylococcus aureus*. Fungal agents such as *Aspergillus niger* and *Candida albicans* may be present along with bacteria or as the sole infecting agent.

A *localized abscess* (*furuncle*) of a hair follicle in the outer two thirds of the ear canal can cause localized external otitis. These small abscesses, caused by minor trauma such as induced by a fingernail in the canal, usually contain *Staphylococcus aureus*.

Viral external otitis occurs frequently. *Herpes zoster* external otitis (Ramsay Hunt syndrome) presents with external ear and oropharyngeal vesicles and may cause facial nerve paralysis, hearing loss, and vestibular dysfunction on the same side. Chickenpox (*varicella*) and *Herpes hominis* may involve the external ear and canal.

Any of these infections, which occur most commonly in the external ear canal, can spread to involve the auricle with the inflammatory process. Cellulitis of the pinna must be treated promptly with systemic antibiotics to prevent perichondritis with necrosis of the auricular cartilage.

Diagnosis

External otitis may present with sensations of mild itching, fullness in the ear, or a severe throbbing pain. The pain is acutely exacerbated when the ear canal is manipulated by opening and closing the jaw or touching the pinna. This response is helpful in distinguishing external otitis from acute otitis media (in which touching the pinna and chewing cause no increased discomfort). Discharge is usually present and may range from a scant watery drainage to one that is profuse, thick, and obviously purulent. Fever is rarely present in the external otitis unless the infection has spread to cause local tissue cellulitis, regional cervical adenitis, or both.

In external otitis, the external meatus is inflamed and swollen. If a furuncle is present, the swelling may be localized to one area, but if the infection is diffuse, the entire circumference of the canal is affected. The canal can be so edematous that the meatus may appear closed. There may also be cellulitis of the surrounding tissues and regional cervical adenitis. Otoscopic examination requires manipulation of the pinna and, therefore, causes severe pain. Visualization of the tympanic membrane may be difficult or impossible if the edema of the canal is very severe or the canal is filled with secretions. Clearing the canal of secretions, should be performed to determine the presence of a normal, intact tympanic membrane in order to rule out acute otitis media and to confirm external otitis as the source of the ear canal discharge.

Complications

The swelling of the ear canal and retention of purulent debris in external otitis cause a mild conductive hearing loss that resolves completely as the infection subsides. Permanent changes in the ear canal may occur as a result of external otitis. The ear canal skin is more susceptible to reinfection for a period of several weeks following an infection. Repeated bouts of external otitis can cause hypertrophy of the subcutaneous tissues and fibrosis of the ear canal, leading to severe narrowing or stenosis of the ear canal.

Malignant external otitis is a disorder that has only recently been described as occurring in children. It is usually seen in children who are severely ill or who have congenital or acquired (chemotherapy, diabetes) immune-deficiency states. In these cases, cellulitis of the ear canal can become extensive, causing necrosis of the auricle, facial nerve paralysis, and mastoid osteomyelitis.

Treatment

In external otitis, as in many situations, prevention is the best treatment. Particular attention should be directed toward preventing the occurrence of any conditions that predispose to external otitis. Maceration, instrumentation, and foreign bodies in the ear canal should be avoided. Prophylactic use of a dilute solution of acetic acid and alcohol drops (prepared by a 1:1 solution of vinegar and alcohol) is often effective in preventing external otitis in children at risk for infection (e.g., competitive swimmers).

Treatment of external otitis requires prompt topical antibiotic therapy as well as attention to any predisposing condition; for instance, swimming should be stopped, and any foreign bodies should obviously be removed. Essential to the rapid resolution of the diffuse external otitis is careful and effective cleaning of the ear canal. Foreign bodies, wax, and purulent material should be cleared from the canal with the appropriate instruments. This not only removes infecting debris, but also clears a path to permit entry of topical antibiotic eardrops effective against organisms commonly found in external otitis. These drops often contain topical corticosteroids to hasten the resolution of inflammation, edema, and pain. Acetic acid drops are also effective in treating external otitis but appear to be most useful when fungi are the infecting organisms. These drops have the added advantage of restoring the normal acid pH to the ear canal, which tends to inhibit external otitis. Nystatin cream placed in the ear canal can also be effective against fungi.

Occasionally the ear canal is so swollen that eardrops cannot enter. A wick of cotton, plain gauze or sponge, should be inserted gently into the canal to facilitate the entrance of the drops by capillary action. The wick should be removed and a new one reinserted, if necessary, in 24 to 48 hours. As the edema subsides, the canal will open and permit entrance of the antibiotic drops without the necessity of the wick. In cases of localized external otitis, any pustule that is pointing should be nicked and opened with the point of an 18-gauge needle. If the external otitis has spread to involve the auricle or regional lymph nodes, a course of broad-spectrum systemic antibiotics should be instituted. In severe cases, the intravenous medications may be necessary. Narcotic analgesic medications may be required for intense pain.

Medical treatment of malignant external otitis *requires intravenous systemic antibiotics effective against Pseudomonas and Staphylococcus* aureus. Surgical drainage of the ear and mastoid is essential to prevent severe morbidity and mortality.

There is no treatment for viral external otitis except to provide symptomatic relief. The pain of *Herpes zoster oticus* is especially severe, and pain relief afforded by narcotic medication is greatly appreciated.

Children with external otitis should be referred to an otolaryngologist when the infection is severe or refractory to conventional therapy. Cleansing of the external canal or surgical drainage may be required to clear the infection.

LABYRINTHITIS (VESTIBULAR AND COCHLEAR)

Serous labyrinthitis is a sterile inflammatory condition characterized by mild vertigo without sensorineural hearing loss. The condition usually occurs when there is inflammation in the adjacent middle ear from either acute or chronic otitis media. The inner ear inflammation and the vertigo resolve as the acute condition subsides. A wide myringotomy may be helpful in these cases. Bacterial labyrinthitis occurs when organisms are actually present in the inner ear. These organisms may enter the inner ear by local spread from an acute otitis media through the oval or round window hematogenously from a distant infection. If this occurs, severe vertigo and a profound sensorineural hearing loss results.

Bacterial labyrinthitis requires antibiotic therapy, wide myringotomy, and possible surgical drainage of the labyrinth to avoid intracranial spread of the infection. As the infection is treated, the vertigo will stabilize and will usually disappear completely within weeks. Any sensorineural hearing loss caused by the bacterial labyrinthitis is usually permanent.

Viral infection of the *labyrinth* may occur, usually in association with an upper respiratory tract infection. The resultant dizziness may be constant or episodic. The one feature helpful in distinguishing viral labyrinthitis from one of the bacterial origin is that the viral form is generally not associated with sensorineural hearing loss. The vertigo usually resolves within several weeks.

Some viral infections of the inner ear may affect the cochlea without causing vertigo. Measles and mumps infections may cause a unilateral or bilateral severe sensorineural deafness. Prenatal infection with cytomegalovirus and rubella can also cause profound deafness. Viral cochleitis is one of the causes of sudden hearing loss in children. Sudden hearing loss without any other associated symptom is the mode of presentation of this entity. While occasionally there is some recovery of hearing in these patients, the hearing loss is usually permanent.

NEOPLASMS

Fortunately, neoplasms of the external ear are rare in young patients. However, one must be watchful of skin and pigment changes that can indicate the presence of a *squamous cell carcinoma* or *malignant melanoma*. Rarely, tumors of the periauricular tissues, such as parotid neoplasms, will invade the ear canal and appear in the external meatus. Management of these neoplasms in children and adolescents is the same as for adults.

Osteomas are the most common benign tumor found in the ear canal and are usually seen in the adolescent or young adult who is a cold water swimmer. Osteomas appear as single or multiple firm, smooth masses in the medial third of the ear canal. They require treatment by surgical removal if they occlude the external canal, causing a hearing loss or recurrent external otitis by retention of moisture and debris.

In the middle ear, benign and malignant tumors are also rarely seen. They present devastating problems because they are usually diagnosed after symptoms have been present for months. *Glomus jugulare* or *glomus tympanicum* (chemodectomas) usually present in the lower half of the middle ear as a pulsatile red mass pushing against the ear drum. Tinnitus synchronous with the patient's pulse is characteristic of these vascular tumors. As the tumor enlarges, it can perforate the tympanic membrane and cause hemorrhage otorrhea. Facial nerve paralysis, vertigo, and sensorineural hearing loss may develop as well.

Rhabdomyosarcoma, lymphoma, or *eosinophilic granuloma* may appear in the middle ear as a fleshy mass of granular friable tissue or edematous polypoid mucosa extending through a tympanic membrane perforation. Since these malignant tumors grow from within the temporal bone, facial nerve paralysis and intracranial spread may occur early in the course of disease. Sensorineural deafness and vestibular dysfunction are also common. The middle ear (like the external canal) may be involved by local spread of tumor from the parotid gland or the nasopharynx (via the eustachian tube).

Primary tumors of the inner ear are rare, but intracranial and metastatic tumors may involve the temporal bone and mastoid. A *schwannoma* is a benign tumor that can occur in the internal auditory canal of children and adolescents. This tumor usually originates in the vestibular division of the eighth cranial nerve but often expands, compressing the cochlear division and causing progressive vertigo and sensorineural deafness. It is most commonly seen in patients with neurofibromatosis and is often bilateral, but it may occur unilaterally in otherwise normal children. A CT scans demonstrates the expansion of the internal auditory canal as a result of tumor growth. Surgical removal is the treatment of choice for these benign lesions.

Early recognition of these lesions is mandatory to ensure proper treatment and maximal survival. Any patients with an external canal or middle ear mass should be referred to an otolaryngologist for evaluation, possible biopsy, and treatment. Similarly, any child with an ear infection that does not respond to appropriate conventional management should be seen by an otolaryngologist, as the infection may be the first sign of an unsuspected ear neoplasm.

TRAUMA

External Ear

External ear trauma is common because the pinna is in an exposed position on the side of the head. Reflex turning of the face to the side to avoid a blow places the ear directly in the line of injury. Blunt trauma to the auricle is common in children and adolescents during a fall or athletic activity. Blunt trauma may cause rupture of small blood vessels, producing ecchymosis of the soft tissue, or it may result in disruption of the perichondrial blood supply, resulting in the formation of a hematoma or seroma. Hematomas and seromas appear as smooth masses on the surface of the ear that obscure the normal auricular contour.

Prevention of ear trauma is important in children who are potentially susceptible to these injuries. Wrestlers and children with poor neuromuscular or head control should wear head or ear protectors. Lacerations and abrasions of the auricle or canal should be treated with local and systemic

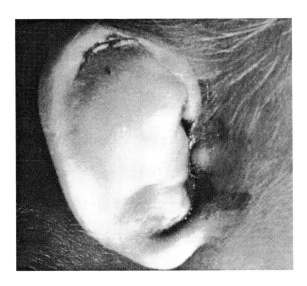

Figure 1–13. Auricular hematoma.

care as necessary. (See the section on foreign bodies for further discussion of ear canal injuries.) Auricular hematomas and seromas (Fig. 1-13) should be drained as soon as possible to prevent permanent cosmetic deformity to the pinna.

The blood supply to the ear originates from the base, leaving the major portions of the pinna surrounded by air. This makes the ear vulnerable to cold injury (frostbite) and burns. These injuries are discussed in the section of thermal injuries.

Tympanic Membrane and Middle Ear

Occasionally, blunt trauma to the head, such as a slap, is sufficient to perforate the tympanic membrane, but most often perforation is caused by a penetrating foreign body. Most traumatic perforations of the tympanic membrane heal completely and without complication in less than six weeks, provided that infection is prevented and the edges of the perforation are not folded inward into the middle ear. All children with traumatic perforations should be examined by an otolaryngologist to be certain that epithelium is not folded into the ear, setting the stage for cholesteatoma formation. A 10-day course of oral antibiotics, usually penicillin, is given to prevent infection. However, if the middle ear was contaminated during the injury (e.g., in a swimming pool), antibiotic otic drops are also recommended. When facial nerve paralysis or perilymph fistula occurs with a traumatic perforation of the tympanic membrane, immediate middle ear exploration of the injury is required for proper treatment. Uncomplicated perforations that do not heal within six weeks and any ossicular disruption can be repaired electively.

The structures in the middle ear may be damaged with or without disruption of the tympanic membrane and result in ossicular dislocation, facial nerve paralysis, or fracture of the stapes footplate and perilymph fistula. Blunt trauma to the head produces shearing forces that may disrupt the middle ear mucosa, resulting in bleeding into the middle ear space (hemotympanum). Barotrauma during airplane flight or underwater activities may also cause hemotympanum. The diagnosis is made by pneumatic otoscopy while tympanoplasty can confirm the presence of fluid in the middle ear. Blood and serous fluid usually clear from the middle ear within a few days following barotrauma or blunt head injury. Antibiotics are not usually administered in these cases but are useful to prevent secondary infection. However, when a hearing loss and effusion remain two to four weeks after middle ear trauma, the patient should be referred to an otolaryngologist for possible myringotomy and insertion of a ventilation tube.

It should be remembered that perilymph fistula and ossicular discontinuity may occur behind an intact tympanic membrane. The primary care physician must keep this in mind when treating children with middle ear trauma.

Inner Ear

Blunt head trauma of insufficient force to fracture the skull can disrupt the tissue integrity of the cochlear and vestibular labyrinth. Hemorrhage may occur in the labyrinth (hemorrhage labyrinthitis) and produce sensorineural hearing loss and vertigo.

Temporal bone fractures most often occur in conjunction with more extensive fractures of the base of the skull. As many as 80% of temporal bone fractures occur along the long axis of the petrous bone. These longitudinal fractures frequently cause bloody cerebrospinal fluid otorrhea through a disrupted tympanic membrane, ossicular discontinuity, and facial nerve paralysis that is either immediate or delayed in onset. Transverse fractures are associated with hemotympanum (blood behind an intact tympanic membrane) and inner ear damage (sensorineural hearing loss and vertigo). No attempt should be made by the primary care physician to clear the blood from the ear canal of a patient with a temporal bone fracture. Manipulation may introduce organisms into the middle ear and possibly into the cranium, resulting in meningitis. Facial nerve function should be noted and recorded. Delayed or partial facial paralysis will usually resolve over a period of several weeks, but immediate total paralysis requires early facial nerve exploration and repair of the damaged nerve. Systemic antibiotics should be given until the cerebrospinal fluid otorrhea subsides, usually within a few days. Persistent cerebrospinal fluid otorrhea, conductive hearing loss, or perforation of the tympanic membrane will require surgical repair. All patients with a temporal bone fracture should be referred to an otolaryngologist.

Barotrauma, blunt head injuries, or straining during physician exertion can cause a perilymph fistula or leak of perilymph through the oval or round window. Sudden hearing loss and constant or fluctuating vertigo are the signs of a perilymph fistula. These patients should be referred to an otolaryngologist for evaluation and possible middle ear exploration to plug the leak.

Thermal Injury

Thermal injury to the ear may result from exposure to extremes in temperature. Cold thermal injury is obviously most common in cold climates. Burn injuries may result from excessive sun (rarely) and from fire exposure. Thermal injury from cold (frostbite) and heat (burns) can be classified in a similar matter (Table 1-3).

First-degree burns require little treatment. The injured skin should be dressed with a mild antibiotic ointment. All children with second- and third-degree burns should be seen by an otolaryngologist. No dressing or ointment should be applied to the ear. The consulting otolaryngologist will direct treatment to preserve auricular tissue, encourage reepithelization,

TABLE 1-3 Thermal Injury

Degree of Injury	Burn or Frostbite
First	Erythema of the skin
Second	Bulla (blister) formation
Third	Full-thickness skin loss
Fourth	Loss of auricular tissue (skin and cartilage)

and prevent immediate and delayed infection that could result in perichondritis and cartilage necrosis.

Frostbite injury should be suspected when an auricle is cold, pale, and painful on rewarming. The ear should be rewarmed rapidly by applying wet cotton pledgets soaked in 38 to 42° C saline. Care should be taken to avoid added injury by excessive manipulation. The ear should be completely thawed and not recooled. The rapid rewarming process can be painful; narcotic analgesics and sedatives may be required for comfort. First-degree frostbite requires no further treatment. More extensive injury will require otolaryngologic evaluation and treatment as outlined above.

Foreign Bodies

Foreign bodies of the ear canal are frequently encountered in children. There may be a history of the child or a playmate placing the object in the ear, or the foreign body may be found during a routine otoscopic examination. Attention may be drawn to the ear when infection develops around the material in the ear canal causing pain and discharge. Stones, toys, food (beans, nuts), paper, and occasionally insects are found in the ear canal.

Foreign bodies should be removed in a safe manner as promptly as possible. The method used to remove a foreign body is best determined by the shape and position of the material. Irregular foreign bodies often present an edge than can be grasped using a fine ear forceps. Round foreign bodies, such as beads, are difficult to grasp. A foreign body lying in the outer two thirds of the ear canal should be gently rolled or scooped to the external meatus, where it can be extracted easily (Fig. 1-14). Constant gentle pressure should be maintained against the foreign body to prevent it from falling deeper into the ear as the curette is withdrawn. Care should also be taken to avoid trauma to the surrounding ear canal skin and tympanic membrane. If a round foreign object is in the medial one third of the canal and against the tympanic membrane, the curette should not be used because of the likelihood of trauma to the tympanic membrane. Irrigation with room temperature water directed along the posterior portion of the canal will usually bring the foreign body to the lateral two thirds of the canal, where it will fall out or permit easy removal with a curette (*see* Fig. 1-5).

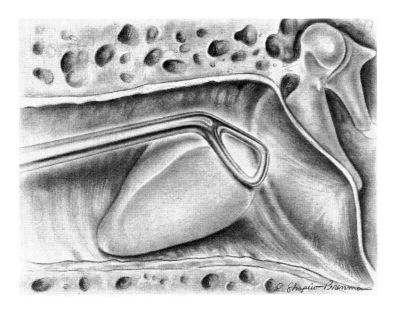

Figure 1–14. Ear curette is used to remove a foreign body (kernel of corn) from the external ear canal.

Insects should be killed by filling the meatus with ether, lidocaine, mineral oil, or alcohol before removal is attempted. Once the insect is dead, it can be easily removed with a forceps.

After a foreign body has been removed, the ear canal must be carefully examined for evidence of trauma or infection. Perforations of the tympanic membrane must be detected. Small lacerations, abrasions, or tympanic membrane perforations will usually heal without treatment. If infection is present in the ear canal, antibiotic containing eardrops should be used for 10 days.

If the removal of a foreign body in the ear canal would be difficult to achieve without causing severe pain or if it is likely to produce significant injury to the ear, the patient should be referred to an otolaryngologist. Similarly, if adequate instruments are not available, if blood becomes evident during attempted removal, or if the child is uncooperative, an otolaryngologist should be consulted. In many of these complicated situations, a general anesthetic may be required to remove the foreign body safely with a minimum of physical and psychological damage to the child.

SUGGESTED READINGS

Bergstrom L, Hemenway WG, Downs MP: A high risk registry to find congenital deafness. *Otolaryngol Clin North Am* 4:369, 1971.

Bluestone CD, Klein JO: Otitis Media in Infants and Children. Philadelphia, W. B. Saunders Co., 1988.

Bluestone CD, Klein, JO: Otitis media, atelectasis and eustachian tube dysfunction. In: Bluestone CD and Stool DE (eds): Pediatric Otolaryngology, 2nd Ed. Philadelphia, W. B. Saunders Co., 1990. pp. 320-486.

Dobie RA, Berlin CI: Influence of otitis media on hearing and development. *Ann Otol Rhinol Laryngol* 88 (Supp 60): 48-53, 1979.

Friedmann I, Arnold W: Pathology of the Ear. New York, Churchill Livingstone, 1993.

Gates GA: Acute otitis media and otitis media with effusion. In: Cummings CW, et al (eds): Otolaryngology-Head and Neck Surgery. St. Louis, Mosby, 1993. pp. 2808-2822.

Gates GA, Avery CA, Cooper JC, Jr, Prihoda TJ: Chronic secretory otitis media: Effects of surgical management. *Ann Otol Rhinol Laryngol* (Supp):138:2-32, 1989.

Konigsmark BW, Gorlin RJ: Genetic and Metabolic Deafness. Philadelphia, W. B. Saunders Co., 1976.

Mandel EM, Rockette HE, Bluestone CD, Paradise JL, Nozza RJ: Efficacy of amoxicillin with and without decongestant-antihistamine for otitis media with effusion in children: Results of a double-blind randomized trial. *N Engl J Med* 316:432-437, 1987.

Niederman LG, Walter-Bucholtz V, Jabalay T: A comparative trial of steroids versus placebos for treatment of chronic otitis media with effusion. In: Proceedings of the 4th International Symposium on Recent Advances in Otitis Media. Burlington, Ontario, B. C. Decker, Inc. 1984. pp. 273-275.

Potsic WP: Management of trauma of the external ear. In: English G (ed): Otolaryngology. Hagerstown, Harper and Row, Vol. 4, Chap. 14. pp. 1-11, 1980.

Proctor CA, Proctor B: Understanding hereditary nerve deafness. *Arch Otolaryngol* 85:45, 1967.

Roland PS, Finitzo T, Friel-Patti S, et al: Otitis media: Incidence, duration and hearing status. *Arch Otolaryngol Head Neck Surg* 115(9):1049-1053, 1989.

Rosenfeld RM, Post JC: Meta-analysis of antibiotics for the treatment of otitis media with effusion. *Otolaryngol Head Neck Surg* 106:378-386, 1992.

Sando I, Wood RP: Congenital middle ear anomalies. *Otolaryngol Clin North Am* 4:291, 1971.

Teele DW, Klein JO, Rosner B: Epidemiology of otitis media during the first seven years of life in children in Greater Boston: A prospective cohort study. *J Infect Diseases* 160(1):83-94, 1989.

CHAPTER 2

NOSE AND
PARANASAL SINUSES

ANATOMY

For ease of discussion, the nose is commonly divided into an external and an internal portion. The external nose (Fig. 2-1) is the visible part that is most susceptible to trauma; it consists of a skin covering over a framework of bone and cartilage. The skin of the nose is loosely attached to the nasal bones but is more firmly adherent to the paired cartilages.

The internal nasal cavity is divided into right and left halves by the nasal septum. The septum extends from the columella posteriorly to the nasopharynx and from the palate upward to the roof of the nose or cribriform plate (Fig. 2-2). It consists of cartilage anteriorly and of bone posteriorly. Minor deflections of the septum into one or both nasal cavities are very common. The nasal cavities extend from the nares (nostrils) anteriorly to the choanae (opening into the nasopharynx) posteriorly. The lateral walls of the nose contain three mucosal-covered scroll-shaped bony projections, the inferior, middle, and superior turbinates. Between the turbinates are recesses, or meatus, into which adjacent structures drain; the nasolacrimal duct (inferior meatus); the frontal, maxillary, and anterior ethmoid sinuses (middle meatus); and the sphenoid and posterior ethmoid sinuses (superior meatus). The nasal cavities are lined with cili-

59

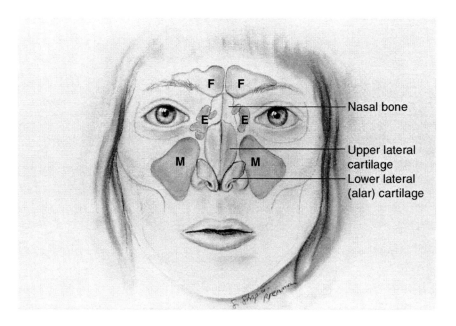

Figure 2–1. Frontal view of face demonstrating paranasal sinuses and skeletal support of external nose. F= Frontal sinuses; E = Ethmoid sinuses; M= Maxillary sinuses.

ated mucus-secreting epithelium. Specialized olfactory epithelium at the roof of the nose is in contact with the olfactory bulb through numerous neural fibers traversing the cribriform plate.

The paranasal sinuses consist of the maxillary, ethmoid, frontal, and sphenoid sinuses (Fig. 2-1). The maxillary and ethmoid sinuses are present at birth. The frontal and sphenoid sinuses appear late and do not reach full development until adolescence. These air-filled spaces communicate with, and almost completely surround, the nasal cavities. They are lined with respiratory epithelium similar to that found in the nose. The maxillary sinuses are present on either side of the interior half of the nose and below the orbits. The buds for the deciduous and permanent teeth are found in the floor of the sinuses (formed by the maxillary alveolar ridge and hard plate) and in the anterior wall. A single large ostium in the middle meatus of the nose drains each maxillary sinus; accessory ostia are occasionally found as well.

The ethmoid sinuses are a cluster or labyrinth of air cells located between each orbit and the upper half of the nasal cavity. Their superior boundary is the cribriform plate, or floor of the anterior cranial fossa. They drain through multiple ostia in the middle meatus (anterior ethmoid cells) and the superior meatus (posterior ethmoid cells).

The frontal sinus is contained within the frontal bone and is located above the nose and orbits. Posteriorly, it is separated from the anterior cranial fossa by a bony wall. The frontal sinus is of variable size and configuration; it is divided into right and left portions by a septum. A nasofrontal duct drains each side into the nose under its respective middle turbinate.

The sphenoid sinus is a midline structure found within the sphenoid bone. The floor of the sphenoid sinus forms the roof of nasopharynx. It is bounded on either side by the cavernous sinus containing its associated neural and vascular structures. The roof of the sphenoid sinus is the sella turcica,

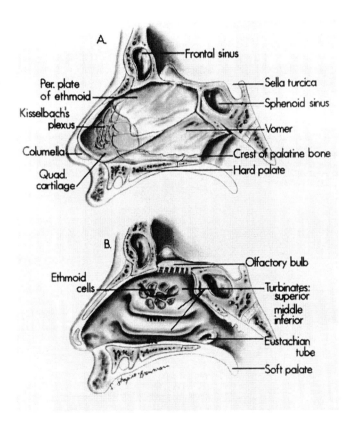

Figure 2–2. Internal nasal cavity. (**A**) Septum. (**B**) Lateral wall of the nose (ethmoid sinuses are lateral to the middle and superior turbinates). mm = middle meatus; im = inferior meatus. (From Potsic WP, Handler SD, Wetmore RF: Ear, Nose, Throat and Mouth. In: Rudolph A (ed). Pediatrics. 19th ed. Norwalk, CT, Appleton & Lange, 1991.)

which contains the pituitary glands. A septum often divides the sinus into two parts, each draining through and ostium into the nasopharynx above its respective superior turbinate.

The blood supply to the nose and paranasal sinuses is complex and derives from both internal and external carotid systems. The rich plexus of anastamoses between these arterial systems results in a blood supply of great variability. A prominent plexus of vessels on the anterior-inferior septum (Little's or Kiesselbach's area) is the most common site of epistaxis in children.

The nerve supply to the nose and paranasal sinuses consists of sensory branches from the first and second divisions of the fifth cranial nerve. Autonomic innervation reaches this area through the vidian nerve, carrying sympathetic fibers derived from the carotid sympathetic chain, and through the parasympathetic fibers from the greater superficial petrosal nerve, a branch of the seventh cranial nerve. Sensory fibers originating in the specialized olfactory epithelium at the roof of the nose perforate the cribriform plate to form the olfactory bulb of the first cranial nerve.

PHYSIOLOGY

Respiration

The nose and paranasal sinuses perform several functions; the first of which involves the process of respiration. The nasal cavities filter the inspired air and regulate its humidity and temperature. The turbinates serve to increase the surface area of the mucus-secreting epithelium to facilitate these functions. In the submucosal layers, an abundant plexus of capillaries permits efficient transfer of heat and water, keeping the air that reaches the nasopharynx at a constant temperature and humidity despite wide fluctuations in the inspired air. Normal nasal breathing occurs primarily through only one side of the nose at a time, switching from one side to the other many times during the day. This nasal cycle is the result of periodic engorgement of blood vessels, decreasing the lumen on that side of the nose. Breathing occurs through the other, less congested, side. The site of nasal respiration alternates in cycles of two to seven hours. The significance of this nasal cycle and the precise mechanism regulating its control are unknown.

Large foreign particles are trapped by the nasal hairs or vibrissae at the entrance of the nose. Smaller particles are caught on the mucus blanket produced by the secretory cells of the respiratory epithelium; this mucus blanket is propelled posteriorly by the beating cilia to the nasopharynx, where it is swallowed.

The precise relationship between the nose and the lower respiratory tract in the control of respiration is controversial. Despite good evidence for the existence of nasopulmonary reflexes, the nature and significance of these interactions are unclear.

The neonate is an obligate nose-breather. The relatively high position of the larynx in the neonate brings the palate into contact with the anterior surface of the epiglottis, effectively sealing off the mouth from the nasal cavities and thereby enabling nasal respiration and suckling to occur simultaneously. As the infant grows, the larynx descends and permits respiration to occur through the nose and mouth.

Olfaction

The olfactory function of the nose is achieved by recognition of the size, shape, and molecular composition of minute amounts of aromatic compounds. Fibers of the first cranial nerve originate in the specialized sensory epithelium at the roof the nose, pass through the cribriform plate, and terminate in the olfactory centers in the brain.

Speech

Speech production is affected by the configuration and functional status of the nose and the paranasal sinuses. These structures provide a resonance cavity for the production of normal speech. If the nose and sinuses are closed off from the oral cavity as a result of choanal atresia or adenoid hypertrophy, for instance, the voice is hyponasal. If the child's nose communicates freely with the oral cavity, as in cleft palate or velopharyngeal insufficiency, the voice will be hypernasal.

Sinuses

The precise function of the paranasal sinuses is unknown, but it has been suggested that they serve to lighten the solid bones of the skull, a possible factor that led to man's erect posture. The sinuses also serve as additional resonance cavities in the production of speech. The sinuses are lined with ciliated, mucus-secreting respiratory epithelium similar to that found in the nasal cavity. The cilia move the sinus mucus blanket of as much as 1 liter/day to the sinus ostia and out into the nose. Obstruction of the ostia by tumor, polyp, or mucosal edema will lead to fluid retention in the affected sinus. If this fluid becomes secondarily infected, acute sinusitis will result.

METHODS OF EXAMINATION

Direct and Indirect Examination

The external nose and anterior potion of the nasal cavities can be examined by direct visual inspection. A nasal speculum and directed light source facilitate visualization of the anterior septum and inferior and middle turbinates. In younger children, the examiner's thumb can elevate the mobile nasal tip so that the anterior nasal structures can be examined (Fig. 2-3). Vasoconstrictors such as phenylephrine can be applied to the nose to shrink the mucosa and permit a more complete examination. The posterior nasal structures and nasopharynx can be seen with the aid of a nasopharyngeal mirror or a fiberoptic telescope placed in either the nose of the posterior oropharynx. Patency of the

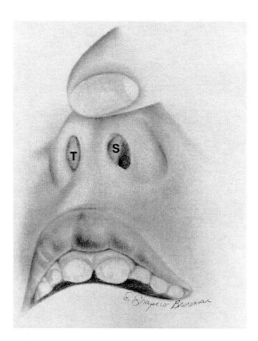

Figure 2–3. Elevation of the nasal tip by the examiner's thumb will usually permit adequate visualization of the anterior nasal structures. T= inferior turbinate; S = septum.

nasal cavities in the neonate can be assessed by the passage of small rubber catheters through the nose and into the pharynx.

Palpation is also important in the examination of the nose and sinuses. Irregularities of the nasal bones, such as fractures or deviation, as well as nasal masses can be detected in this manner. Tenderness to palpation over the sinuses is a common sign of acute sinusitis. Careful examination of adjacent area, including the teeth and orbit, is crucial to the evaluation of sinus disease.

Transillumination of the maxillary sinus can be performed by placing a small penlight in the child's mouth, whose lips are then closed around it. In a dark room, the light should be transmitted equally through the maxillary sinuses to both anterior cheeks. Inequality of the transmitted light indicates a difference in aeration of the sinus, but this nonspecific finding could be caused by fluid, a mass lesion, or hypoplasia of a maxillary sinus. Radiographic techniques, which have largely replaced transillumination in the evaluation of sinus disease, must be used to confirm the specific diagnosis.

Radiologic Examination

Traditionally, plain radiographs have been the radiographic procedure of choice for the evaluation of facial trauma or sinus infection. Computer tomography has now replaced the plain radiograph for most nasal conditions because of its three dimensional views and precise detail. Plain radiographs are still helpful in evaluating the progress of medical therapy in children with sinusitis. CT, however, demonstrates the ostiomeatal complex, the opening between the maxillary sinus and the nasal cavity and the site of most sinus drainage problems. CT is also essential in the evaluation of masses of the nose and sinuses and congenital malformations, such as choanal atresia.

COMMON COMPLAINTS

Rhinorrhea (Runny Nose)

The normal amount of mucus produced by the secreting epithelium of the nose and paranasal sinuses is estimated to be as much as 1000 ml/day. This mucus blanket is swept posteriorly by the cilia into the nasopharynx, where it is swallowed. Anything that increased the amount of mucus production or that interferes with its posterior movement will produce rhinorrhea.

The most frequently seen rhinorrhea is the thin, watery fluid characteristic of the common cold or viral upper respiratory infection. Other signs and symptoms of an upper respiratory infection (fever, malaise, cough, headache) are often present and assist the physician in identifying the cause of the rhinorrhea. A thick yellow-green discharge, especially when associated with systemic symptoms of fever and malaise, usually indicates the presence of acute bacterial infection of the nose or the paranasal sinuses. Typically, there is pain or tenderness over the infected region. Gram-stained fluid will often exhibit many polymorphonuclear leukocytes as well as the causative organisms.

The rhinorrhea associated with an allergic diathesis is often thin and watery. Nasal congestion and other signs and symptoms of nasal allergy often accompany the rhinorrhea. Wright's-stained nasal secretions generally exhibit many eosinophils and a paucity of polymorphonuclear leukocytes.

A clear, watery discharge may indicate cerebrospinal fluid rhinorrhea. The finding of cerebrospinal fluid would indicate an abnormal communication between the intracranial cavity and the nose. While leaks can be caused by hydrocephalus, intracranial tumors, cysts, and congenital malformations such as encephaloceles, the most common cause of cerebrospinal fluid rhinorrhea is trauma. These leaks may occur through the cribriform plate, ethmoid, sinus, frontal sinus, or, less commonly, through the sphenoid sinus and the middle ear. Cerebrospinal fluid rhinorrhea should be suspected in a patient who has a profuse nasal discharge and a history of antecedent trauma. The leak may occur immediately or be delayed for days or even years. Otolaryngologic consultation should be obtained to assist in the investigation of recurrent or persistent rhinorrhea suspicious of a cerebrospinal fluid leak.

Obstruction to the normal posterior mucus flow can lead to an increase in the amount of clinically apparent rhinorrhea. Nasal septal deviation, turbinate hypertrophy, nasal and nasopharyngeal tumors, foreign bodies, adenoid hypertrophy, and choanal atresia can all impede or block the normal mucus flow, producing rhinorrhea. Stasis of these secretions can result in a secondary bacterial infection, with the rhinorrhea showing the characteristic change to a thick, yellow-green secretion. Persistent unilateral purulent rhinorrhea in a child over one year of age, especially if malodorous, should be attributed to a foreign body of the nose until proved otherwise. Unilateral rhinorrhea in a child under one year of age is more likely related to unilateral choanal atresia. If purulent rhinorrhea does not clear up or recurs immediately after appropriate antimicrobial treatment, sinus radiographs should be obtained and the patient referred to an otolaryngologist for a complete examination of the nose, paranasal sinuses, and nasopharynx.

Closely related to the condition of rhinorrhea is that of postnasal or sinus drip. The nasal and sinus mucus normally moves posteriorly into the nasopharynx, where it is swallowed. This process usually occurs unconsciously, but the child may become aware of this process when the secretions increase, as in acute or allergic rhinitis, or when the secretions change in consistency or composition, as in instances of bacterial rhinosinusitis. The patient notices that he has to swallow frequently or that he has to make a conscious effort to swallow particularly tenacious or bad-tasting secretions. This condition is often accompanied by a sore, irritated throat, hoarseness, cough, or a feeling of a lump in the throat. Thick, yellow secretions can often be seen dripping down the posterior oropharynx. Night time cough is an additional symptom, although it may also be associated with cough variant asthma. Auscultation of the chest for expiratory wheezing may distinguish between the two conditions.

Nasal Obstruction (Stuffy Nose)

Obstruction to the normal passage of respiratory gases can occur with a variety of conditions and will give the sensation of a blocked, or stuffy, nose. Temporary partial obstruction of one nasal cavity at a time occurs normally in the nasal cycle. Prolonged blockage, however, is a pathologic condition for which the etiology should be sought. A careful history and examination of the nasal cavities and pharynx (with radiographs as indicated) is necessary to determine the source of the blockage. *Septal deviation, foreign bodies,* and *turbinate hypertrophy* are frequent causes of nasal obstruction. *Nasal tumors* are a rare cause of chronic obstruction. The nasopharynx may be the site of obstruction to nasal airflow. A patient who presents with nasal obstruction could possibly have *adenoid hypertrophy,* a *nasopharyngeal tumor (lymphoma, rhabdomyosarcoma), choanal atresia* (unilateral or bilateral), or a *meningoencephalocele.* If the etiology of the obstruction is not apparent after a careful examination of the nose and nasopharynx, or if the blockage does not respond to conventional medical management, referral should be made to an otolaryngologist. Surgery may be required to extract a foreign body, straighten a deviated nasal septum, biopsy a tumor, or repair the atresia.

Epistaxis (Nosebleed)

While epistaxis is a relatively common occurrence in childhood, it may cause significant anxiety in both the child and the caretaker. Bleeding may occur secondary to the mucosal maceration associated with an upper respiratory infection or as the result of trauma from picking. The usual site of bleeding is the anterior nasal septum, known as Kiesselbach's or Little's area (*see* Fig. 2-2).

A complete history is an important step in the proper management of epistaxis. The site of nasal bleeding (one or both sides of the nose), frequency, presence of bleeding from other sites, history of trauma, and family history of bleeding should be ascertained. Careful examination of the nose should be performed to identify the site and cause of the bleeding. Good lighting, suction, and material for cauterization and packing should be readily available. Topical vasoconstrictors such as phenylephrine can be used to shrink the nasal mucosa to permit better visualization of the nasal cavity and possible slow or even stop the bleeding. Simple pressure exerted by squeezing the nostrils together is usually sufficient to control epistaxis. Occasionally, a roll of cotton placed beneath the upper lip will stop bleeding by compressing the labial artery. If pressure proves unsuccessful, cauterization with silver nitrate sticks or packing of the nose is performed (Fig. 2-4). Absorbable packing such as oxidized cellulose is usually adequate for epistaxis and has the advantage of not having to be removed.

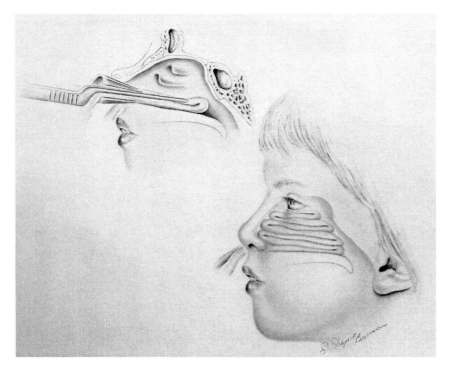

Figure 2–4. Vaseline gauze (1/2 inch wide by 72 inches long) is layered into the nasal cavity to form an anterior nasal pack.

Proper management of severe or recurrent episodes of epistaxis requires the assistance of an otolaryngologist. Epistaxis that fails to stop with simple pressure or absorbable packing may require deeper cauterization or a more substantial anterior nasal pack of Vaseline®-impregnated gauze. A posterior nasal pack, using gauze or a Foley catheter, may rarely be necessary to control epistaxis originating in the posterior nasal cavity or nasopharynx (Fig. 2-5). A child who requires a posterior pack should be hospitalized for observation of any further bleeding and of any airway obstruction secondary to the packing. Treatment of the child with recurrent epistaxis should include measures to prevent traumatizing the nose; otherwise the child might continue to cause further bleeding. A vaporizer placed in the child's room will increase the hu-

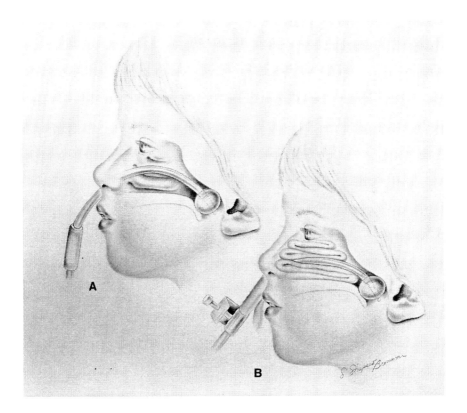

Figure 2–5. Posterior nasal pack. (**A**) A Foley catheter is threaded through the nostril into the nasopharynx. The balloon is inflated and the catheter withdrawn until the balloon is pressed up against the choanae. (**B**) An anterior pack is placed (see Fig. 2-4) and the Foley secured against the pack with a Hoffman C clamp.

midity and thereby soften the nasal mucosa; application of petroleum jelly or antibiotic ointment to the anterior septal areas twice daily can aid in healing the irritated nasal mucosa and prevent recurrent epistaxis. Recurrent or severe bleeding may require cauterization or even ligation of dilated vessels on the septum.

In children with severe or recurrent epistaxis, causes other than simple nose-picking should be ruled out. *Nasal septal deviation* or *perforation, sinusitis, tumor (nasal, nasopharyngeal, or sinus)*, and *nasal foreign body* can all present with epistaxis. Blood dyscrasias such as *hemophilia, idiopathic thrombocytopenia purpura, von Willebrand's disease*, and *hematologic conditions* associated with leukemia or the administration of chemotherapeutic agents may lead to severe epistaxis. Treatment must include the correction of any underlying hematologic problem in addition to the utilization of the previously described local measures. Nasal bleeding is frequently severe in *Osler-Weber-Rendu disease (hereditary hemorrhagic telangiectasia)*, a condition associated with multiple telangiectases throughout the aerodigestive tract. Treatment of the epistaxis associated with this syndrome involves extensive resection of the fragile nasal mucosa and resurfacing of the nasal cavity with skin grafts.

CONGENITAL MALFORMATIONS

Cleft Palate and Lip

The most common congenital malformations of the nose are those associated with *cleft palate* and *lip deformities*. The nasal septum is always deviated in patients with cleft palate as well as in those patients in whom the cleft lip deformity extends into the nasal cavity. The columella may be short, deviated to one side, or even absent, resulting in a nasal tip deformity. Nasal clefts and congenital sinuses can occur as isolated findings or in conjunction with other cleft palate and lip deformities. Craniofacial anomalies such as Apert's, Crouzon's, or Down's syndromes are classically associated with hypoplasia of the maxillary bone, and consequently, of the maxillary sinus.

Choanal Atresia

Since the newborn infant is an obligate nose-breather, bilateral choanal atresia will cause significant respiratory distress at birth. Choanal atresia occurs as a result of failure of breakdown of the buconasal membrane in the six-week-old embryo. The deformity can be bilateral or unilateral (approximately equal occurrence), and more than 90% are bony in nature. Choanal atresia should be suspected in a neonate whose respiratory distress disappears upon opening the mouth to cry. The diagnosis can be confirmed by the failure of nasal catheters or of radiographic contrast material to pass through the nose into the pharynx. Immediate management consists of keeping the infant's mouth open with a large, open nipple (McGovern nipple) or with a large orogastric tube taped or tied in place. As these newborn infants experience significant respiratory problems when attempting to feed, they may require an orogastric tube until they learn to coordinate eating and breathing.

In the past, the management of bilateral choanal atresia was dependent upon the child's age. If the child was feeding well and tolerated a McGovern nipple for breathing, a transnasal repair was performed when the child reached either ten pounds of weight or one year of age.

Experience with the transnasal technique has demonstrated that early repair is preferable. The bony atresia plate is easily perforated in a newborn infant if care is taken to protect the skull base posterior to it. Plastic stents, typically fashioned from a cut endotracheal tube, are left in place for four to six weeks. The infant may require several dilations after the stents are removed.

Some children have difficulty tolerating a McGovern nipple or demonstrate respiratory compromise after a transnasal repair. In such recalcitrant cases, a tracheostomy may be necessary.

In an older child, transnasal repair may be difficult due to the thickness of the bony atresia plate. A transpalatal approach allows the otolaryngologist to drill away this plate under direct vision.

Unilateral choanal atresia seldom causes respiratory distress and may only be detected when evaluating an older child complaining of a persistent unilateral nasal discharge. Repair in an older child involves removal of the posterior nasal septum.

Choanal stenosis can cause respiratory distress, depending on the degree of narrowing. Conservative treatment is recommended with careful nasal suctioning to maintain a patent airway. Otolaryngologic consultation should be sought to assist in calibrating the size of the stenotic nasal passage. Repeated attempts at dilating narrow choanae can worsen the stenosis and cause complete obstruction. Persistent and symptomatic stenosis may require surgical repair similar to that used for patients with choanal atresia.

Congenital Masses

Dermoid cysts are epithelial-lined structures that arise from trapped epithelial rests near lines of embryonic fusion. The midline of the nose, the area be-

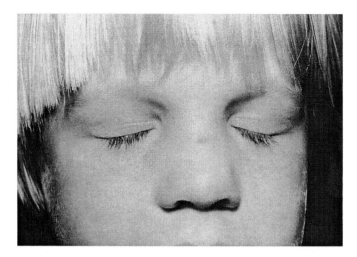

Figure 2–6. Nasal dermoid presenting as a small pit on the dorsum of the nose. (From Potsic WP, Handler SD, Wetmore RF: Ear, Nose, Throat and Mouth. In: Rudolph A (ed). Pediatrics. 19th ed. Norwalk, CT, Appleton & Lange, 1991.)

tween the orbit and the nose, and the lateral supraorbital ridge are common sites of presentation. Nasal dermoids often appear as a pit or swelling on the dorsum of the nose (Fig. 2-6). Other cysts may present in the mouth or on the floor of the nose between the lateral palatal processes (palatine cyst) or between the lip and upper alveolar ridge (nasoalveolar cyst). While these cysts are usually isolated to the nose, occasionally they have an intracranial extension. MR scanning is useful for demonstrating such corrections.

Encephaloceles and *gliomas* are epithelial or glial extensions of the central nervous system, which have passed through the floor of the frontal fossa and appear in or about the nose. Pulsations synchronous with the pulse and that exhibit enlargement when the child is crying indicate that the mass contains cerebrospinal fluid and is in continuity with the central nervous system. An otolaryngologist should be consulted to assist in the evaluation and treatment of these congenital masses. Aspiration or simple excision of these masses is to be avoided because of the danger of cerebrospinal fluid rhinorrhea and subsequent meningitis. A combined otolaryngologic-neurosurgical excision is required for those masses with intracranial extension.

Aplasia or *hypoplasia* of the paranasal sinuses occurs uncommonly in children. Hypoplasia of the maxillary sinus may be an isolated deformity or may be associated with a known craniofacial anomaly such as acrocephalosyndactylia *(Apert's syndrome)* or craniofacial dysostosis *(Crouzon's syndrome)*. Frontal sinuses are absent in up to 4% of otherwise normal people. Most of these congenital anomalies cause no problems.

A *bifid nose*, caused by incomplete fusion of the two nasal placodes, and *absence of the nose* are extremely rare congenital malformations. *Congenital dislocation of the nasal septum*, thought to be caused by birth trauma, is indicated by nasal tip deviation and obstruction at birth.

INFECTIOUS DISEASES

Viral Infections

Viral infections account for most infections of the nose and sinuses in children. The syndrome of fever, nasal congestion, headache, and clear rhinorrhea comprises what is usually known as the *common cold* or *upper respiratory infection*. While nasal and sinus symptoms may predominate in an upper respiratory infection, the infection is usually systemic and involves other areas of the upper respiratory tract, such as the pharynx, larynx, trachea, and bronchi. Many organisms, including *rhinovirus, coronavirus, adenovirus, respiratory syncytial virus*, and *coxsackie virus*, have been identified as causative agents. The infection is usually self-limited and lasts about five to seven days, unless complications occur. Treatment is symptomatic, consisting of rest, antipyretics, and oral antihistamines, and/or decongestants.

Topical decongestants may be used to provide relief of the nasal congestion associated with upper respiratory infection. The relief from congestion afforded by these drugs is only temporary; however, congestion of the nose reoccurs as the topical vasoconstrictor wears off. The use of these medications should be limited to less than four or five days, as chronic use can lead to rhinitis medicamentosa, a condition in which the nasal mucosa undergoes metaplastic changes and becomes chronically thickened. The resulting nasal congestion in such cases is refractory to any medication, and the swollen mucosal tissues persist until the topical drugs are discontinued.

Maceration of nasal mucous membranes from the increased mucus production associated with the viral infection can lead to ulceration and to the possible complication of epistaxis or secondary bacterial infection. Acute or secondary otitis media can also occur in association with a viral rhinitis (see Chapter 1). The acute mucosal edema seen in viral rhinitis can extend into the paranasal sinuses and result in a viral sinusitis. Blockage of the sinus ostia causes retention of mucus in the sinus and gives the feeling of fullness and congestion that often accompanies these viral infections. Whereas viral rhinitis can occur without clinically apparent sinusitis, symptomatic sinusitis is almost always accompanied by rhinitis. Radiographs can usually demonstrate mucosal thickening of the sinus mucosa and, occasionally, air-fluid levels. Treatment of viral sinusitis is the same as that for viral rhinitis, with the possible addition of antimicrobial agents such as amoxicillin to prevent secondary bacterial sinusitis.

Bacterial Infections

Acute bacterial rhinitis or sinusitis can occur as an isolated process, but it is more commonly secondary to some other antecedent condition. A viral upper respiratory infection or adenotonsillitis will often precede an acute bacterial infection of the nose or sinuses, or both. The ethmoid and the maxillary sinuses are the sinuses most frequently affected in children. The organisms most commonly involved include *Diplococcus pneumoniae, Streptococcus species, Staphylococcus aureus, Hemophilus influenzae,* and anaerobic species, such as *Peptostreptococcus, Bacteroides,* and *Fusobacterium.* Symptoms of bacterial rhinosinusitis include fever, mucopurulent nasal (or postnasal) discharge, headache, halitosis, and tenderness over the involved sinuses.

Physical examination of the patient with sinusitis will indicate a mucopurulent nasal discharge, inflamed nasal mucosa, and occasionally, a mucopurulent postnasal drip. Radiographs may demonstrate opacification or air-fluid levels, especially if the films are taken with the patient in the upright position. The upright Waters and Caldwell views are the most useful for detecting sinusitis in children.

Treatment of acute uncomplicated bacterial rhinosinusitis consists of all the measures described for viral rhinosinusitis in addition to the appropriate antimicrobial therapy. Appropriate antibiotic therapy includes amoxicillin clavulanate (Augmentin®), a second or third generation cephalosporin (Ceclor®, Ceftin®) or erythromycin-sulfisoxazole (Pediazole®) for 10 to 14 days. Cultures of the nose or nasopharynx, while not always indicative of the actual organism within the sinuses, may be helpful in some cases. Since the ostium of the maxillary sinus may be closed, functional endoscopic sinus surgery (FESS) may be necessary to provide access to pathogens in the sinus if initial therapy is unsuccessful.

Repeat radiographs of the sinuses should be performed 6 to 10 weeks after the acute episode of sinusitis has subsided to make sure that the affected sinuses have re-aerated and do not demonstrate evidence of chronic changes that could lead to recurrent infections.

Acute sinusitis may lead to complications requiring further intervention. Infections can spread from the ethmoid and, occasionally, the maxillary sinus

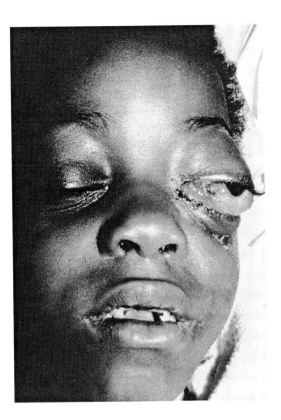

Figure 2–7. Child with orbital abcess as a complication of ethmoid sinusitis. (Photo courtesy of Robert Weisman, MD, University of Pennsylvania.)

into the soft tissues of the orbit, causing either orbital cellulitis or abscess, or both. Proptosis, chemosis, decreased vision and impaired ocular mobility are all signs of orbital involvement with the inflammatory process (Fig. 2-7). The bone and soft tissue overlying the frontal or maxillary sinus may become infected, resulting in osteomyelitis, cellulitis or a subcutaneous abscess of the facial skin. Infections can spread from the ethmoid or frontal sinuses into the intracranial cavity, causing meningitis, epidural abscess, subdural abscess and even brain abscess. Maxillary sinusitis can destroy the tooth buds associated with its anterior and inferior wall and can lead, in rare instances, to an oroantral fistula. Sinus infection can also spread by way of the venous drainage of the face back to the cavernous sinus, resulting in cavernous sinus thrombosis.

When any of the above complications of sinusitis is suspected, the child should be hospitalized immediately for further investigation and treatment. Otolaryngologic consultation should be obtained to assist in the management of the patient. The presence of extrasinus complication may be confirmed by radiographic studies (CT or MRI scans), ophthalmologic consultation and lumbar puncture, if necessary. These patients should be placed on high-dose intravenous antimicrobial therapy. Preferred antibiotic regimes include a combination of oxacillin and either chloramphenicol or a third generation cephalosporin. Medical and surgical therapy depend on the complication and its severity. Mild complications such as periorbital cellulitis usually respond to intravenous antimicrobial therapy within 24 to 48 hours. Failure of resolution or progression of the complication of sinusitis indicates the need for more aggressive intervention. Drainage of the affected sinus, orbital abscess or intracranial abscess may be required, depending on the complication and the sinus involved. The complications of sinusitis should be followed carefully with otolaryngologic, ophthalmologic, neurosurgical, and dental consultations as indicated.

Any child with a complication of sinusitis or with a history of persistent or recurrent sinus infections should be referred to an otolaryngologist for a careful investigation of predisposing conditions. Rhinosinusitis may be the presenting symptom of a nasal foreign body, neoplasm, septal deviation, adenoid hypertrophy, nasal polyp, allergy, abscessed maxillary tooth, or immunodeficiency. Signs and symptoms include chronic purulent rhinorrhea, often with a postnasal drip, as well as headache and nasal congestion. Any child with nasal polyps should be evaluated for cystic fibrosis. Chronic or recurrent sinusitis is associated with Kartagener's syndrome, which consists of situs inversus, sinusitis and bronchiectasis. The diagnosis may be confirmed by the demonstration of abnormal cilia on nasal biopsy. Resolution of the chronic or recurrent sinusitis will depend on elimination or correction of any predisposing conditions.

The organisms obtained in patients with *chronic sinusitis* are usually the same as those seen in acute infections, with the addition of an increased incidence of *Staphylococcus* and anaerobic bacteria. The choice of antibiotic must reflect this expanded range of pathogens. Because it may be difficult to achieve high tissue levels of appropriate antibiotics, treatment periods of four to six weeks are often necessary. Adjunct therapy includes decongestants and topical nasal steroid sprays. If medical therapy fails to resolve the symptoms, CT of the sinuses should be performed. Both axial and coronal sections are necessary to completely visualize all structures. Evidence of blockage of the ostiomeatal complex (the maxillary ostium into the nasal cavity) or the extensive ethmoid sinusitis may require functional endoscopic sinus surgery (FESS) for correction. By using small forceps and suctions under endoscopic guidance, the natural drainage patterns of the nose and sinuses can be established.

Extensive infection in the ethmoid sinuses can be resolved by removal of diseased tissue.

Chronic frontal sinusitis is rare in adolescence, but if present, may necessitate frontal sinus obliteration with abdominal wall fat. Long-standing obstruction of frontal or ethmoidal sinus ostia may result in the accumulation of viscous secretions within the thickened mucosal-lined sinus. The process forms a sac-like structure called a mucocele that slowly expands and erodes adjacent bone through constant pressure. The mucocele may present as an extending mass in either the orbit or cranial cavity. Treatment of a mucocele requires complete excision of the cyst or creation of adequate drainage into the nasal cavity.

Fungal Infections

Fungal infections of the nose and sinus are very uncommon and usually occur in patients with immune-deficiency states. *Aspergillus* and *Candida* species are frequently cultured from the nasal secretions of patients receiving systemic chemotherapy for malignancies. *Mucormycosis* infections are most often seen in young patients with poorly controlled insulin-dependent diabetes mellitus. The classic presentation of this complication is a black, infarcted area of the hard palate or of the lateral nasal wall. Therapy is directed toward correcting the underlying systemic problem while administering systemic and topical antifungal drugs. Local debridement of necrotic tissue is often necessary.

NEOPLASMS

Neoplasms of the nose and sinus are uncommon. They may present as mass lesions or as chronic or recurrent rhinosinusitis. An otolaryngologist should be consulted in the evaluation and treatment of these cases.

Benign Neoplasms

Hemangiomas are the most common neoplasms of the head and neck in children and frequently occur on the skin near or on the nose. Since hemangiomas often go through a period of rapid growth for the first 12 to 18 months of life before beginning to involute, a period of close observation is recommended before any treatment is considered. If the hemangiomas is growing rapidly, causing airway obstruction, thrombocytopenia, high-output cardiac failure, or skin breakdown, early intervention is indicated. Otolaryngologic consultation should be sought to assist the primary practitioner in the management of these difficult problems. Initial treatment with a course of corticosteroids often proves successful in halting the growth of these lesions and can even induce regression. Surgical excision is indicated for those hemangiomas that continue to cause functional or cosmetic deformity after involution has occurred.

Papillomas are viral-induced verrucous growths; they are the most common neoplasms of the aerodigestive tract. When these lesions appear in the nose, they are most often found on the nasal septum. Simple excision or fulguration is the preferred treatment.

Fibro-osseous disorders include *osteomas, giant cell granulomas, fibrous dysplasia, fibroma,* and the *brown tumor of hyperparathyroidism.* After blood tests are performed to rule out hyperparathyroidism, treatment consists of simple excision or sculpturing for cosmetic purposes and for relief of nasal or sinus obstruction.

Malignant Neoplasms

Malignant tumors of the nose and sinuses in children are rare. They include *rhabdomyosarcoma, lymphoma, esthesioneuroblastoma (olfactory esthesioneuroblastoma),* and, rarely, metastatic lesions from primary tumors below the clavicle. These lesions can present with such common symptoms and signs as nasal congestion or epistaxis, with a mass in the nose, or with clinically apparent cervical adenopathy. Treatment usually involves combination therapy with surgery, chemotherapy, and radiotherapy. Since the advent of chemotherapy of the 1960s, survival in children with these tumors has improved significantly.

ALLERGIC CONDITIONS

Manifestations of allergy in the nose and sinuses may range from seasonal bouts of sneezing and rhinorrhea to chronic sinusitis with polyp and mucocele formation. The nose and sinus mucosa are well-known target organs for inhalant and, less frequently, food allergens. Mucosal edema, vascular engorgement, increased numbers of mucous glands, eosinophils, and macrophages can an be present as a result of the actions of vasoactive substances, such as histamine, serotonin, bradykinin, and slow-reacting substance A (SRS-A), released from mast-cell-antibody-antigen complexes. Nasal congestion, watery rhinorrhea, sneezing, and nasal itching are all characteristics of nasal allergy. The rhinorrhea may be seasonal or perennial in nature. Dark circles under the eyes ("allergic shiners") are thought to be caused by allergy-related venous congestions and stasis. The pale bluish tint of the nasal mucosa seen in allergic conditions is believed to be a result of this same venous stasis. A transverse skin crease on the dorsum of the nose is often created by the child's frequent upward wipe — allergic salute — of a constantly runny nose.

While the most important factors in diagnosing nasal allergy are the history and physical examination, laboratory tests such as nasal smear for eosinophils, immunoglobulin E (IgE) levels, and skin testing help confirm the diagnosis and identify the offending allergen. Avoidance of that allergen then becomes the most effective therapy. Hyposensitization, systemic antihistamines, and, occasionally, topical or systemic corticosteroids are also useful in treating the allergy. Nasal polyps, the most commonly seen nasal mass, are almost always a manifestation of nasal allergy in the teenager, although they may be associated with chronic infection or cystic fibrosis in the younger child. Nasal polyps usually originate in the middle turbinate and ethmoid sinus. Antrochoanal polyps originate in the maxillary sinus and extend to the choanae or nasopharynx. An otolaryngologist should be consulted in the treatment of children with nasal polyps, to determine the presence and origin of any polyps as well as perform the surgery necessary to remove the polyps and drain the affected sinuses.

OLFACTORY DISORDERS

Disorders of smell are uncommon in children. Congenital anosmia occurs as an isolated finding or can be associated with hypogonadotrophic hypogonadism (Kallman's syndrome). The most common cause of temporary anosmia is the nasal obstruction associated with an upper respiratory infection. Obstruction of the nasal airway by enlarged adenoids, nasal and nasopharyngeal tumors, or nasal polyps can also cause decreased olfactory function. Trauma (fractures through the cribriform plate), endocrine disorders (Addison's disease, thyroid dysfunction), brain tumors, drugs, viral infections, and exposure to environmental pollutants all affect the child's sense of smell. An otolaryngologist should be sought to determine whether the patient with an olfactory disorder has an intranasal condition responsible for the problem. Radiographs of the nose, paranasal sinuses, and cribriform plate are helpful in the evaluation. However, precise analysis of these disorders is difficult to perform because of the lack of objective and quantitative tests of olfaction. Treatment is directed toward the correction, if possible, of any underlying intranasal or endocrine disorder. If the olfactory epithelium or nerves in the roof of the nose have not sustained irreversible damage, the child's sense of smell may return to normal. The anosmia that results from some viral infections and most frontal cranial trauma is permanent, although some investigators report limited success in the treatment of anosmia or dysosmia with vitamin A.

TRAUMA

Facial trauma occurs frequently in children as a result of play activities, contact sports, and automobile accidents. Several factors help keep these injuries relatively minor in the younger child: (1) younger children are more often involved in low-velocity injuries; (2) they have an increased amount of soft tissue overlying their facial skeletons; and (3) their bony skeletons are less ossified, making a crush or greenstick injury common for this age group. The older child, with increased activities and more rigid skeleton, tends to have more complete fractures.

Any child with facial trauma should undergo careful evaluation to rule out associated cervical, ocular, thoracic, abdominal, and intracranial injuries. Proper management of these serious injuries often takes priority over treatment of the facial injury.

The *nose* is the most frequently injured part of the facial skeleton because of its prominent position on the face and the fragile nature of the nasal bones. A direct blow to the nose can cause lateral deviation or depression of the nasal skeleton and septum. The deformity is usually clinically apparent, although post-injury edema may prevent its recognition for four to five days (Fig. 2-8). Often a stepoff (i.e., bony irregularity) can be palpated, and subcutaneous crepitance may be present. Radiographs of the nose may demonstrate these factors but are of little help in arriving at a suitable course of management. Epistaxis commonly accompanies nasal trauma but usually stops spontaneously. Persistent or severe bleeding may require local pressure, topical vasoconstrictors, or nasal package. Prophylactic antibiotics are commonly given because of the risk of infection in these compound fractures. Ophthalmo-

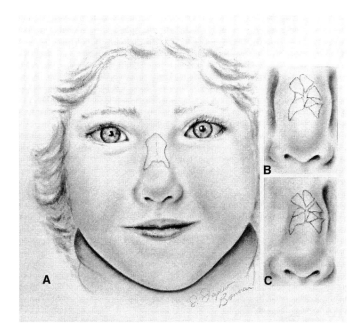

Figure 2–8. Nasal fracture. (**A**) Nasal bones in normal position. (**B**) Marked edema associated with the injury may mask the deviation of nasal bones. (**C**) Deviation of nasal skeleton becomes manifest when edema subsides in approximately three to five days.

logic consultation should be sought to determine the presence of any associated ocular injury, such as hyphema or retinal detachment. In addition, an otolaryngologist should be consulted to confirm whether a nasal fracture has occurred (and the amount of deformity, if any), and to perform any necessary reduction. If a septal hematoma has occurred (Fig. 2-9), it must be recognized and drained promptly with subsequent packing of the mucoperichondrium back against the septal cartilage. Failure to take this step can lead to abscess formation and destruction of the septal cartilage. A saddle nose deformity can result from loss of dorsal support of the external nose. The deviated nose and septum can be reduced under local or general anesthesia once the swelling has subsided enough to permit accurate evaluation of the nasal deformity, usually three to five days. If more than seven days elapse between the time of injury and an attempt at reduction, the fracture fragments will begin to form a strong, fibrous union in their deviated positions, often making reduction impossible. Persistent nasal deformities from unreduced fractures may require rhinoplastic procedures at a later date.

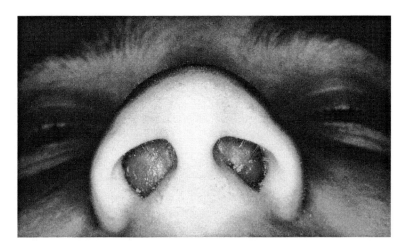

Figure 2–9. Bilateral septal hematoma. (Photo courtesy of Willard Moran, MD, Oklahoma City, Oklahoma. From Handler SD, Wetmore RF: Otolaryngologic Injuries. *Clin Sports Medicine* 1:431-447, 1982.)

Fractures of the facial bones (walls of the paranasal sinuses) may occur as isolated findings or in association with trauma to the nose and the orbital structures. Fractures of the ethmoid sinus or anterior wall of the maxillary sinus usually occur as a result of blunt trauma. Subcutaneous crepitance may be felt in the cheek or around the eye. Radiographs may demonstrate air in the cheek or orbit. The otolaryngologist can assist the primary care physician in evaluating these fractures. After determining the absence of associated ocular injury, the patient is usually placed on oral antibiotics and observed as the crepitance subsides. Surgical intervention is seldom required in the treatment of this condition.

Blunt trauma to the orbit may result in transmission of the force through the globe, breaking the orbital floor (roof of maxillary sinus) or the medial orbital wall (lamina papyracea of the ethmoid sinus). In these *blowout fractures*, orbital fat and muscle can herniate through the bony defect. The patient complains of diplopia (double vision) (Fig. 2-10), and enophthalmos may be evident secondary to the decreased volume of soft tissue within the orbit. Radiographs may reveal the displaced fracture, the presence of orbital contents hanging into the maxillary sinus, or complete opacification of the affected sinus. This injury warrants ophthalmologic consultation, as does any facial injury in which the eye may be affected. If an obvious herniation of orbital contents or if muscle entrapment is detected, reduction of the orbital contents and repair of the fracture site should be performed by an otolaryn-

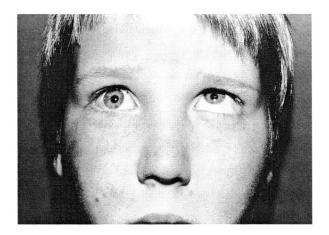

Figure 2–10. Child with right orbital blowout fracture. Diplopia results from inability to elevate right eye on upward gaze.

gologist within five to seven days. If left untreated, this injury can result in permanent diplopia and enophthalmos.

Fractures of the malar bone can occur affecting both the orbital floor and the maxillary sinus. A complete *malar* (incorrectly called *trimalar* or *tripod*) *fracture* is present when the malar bone fractures at the infraorbital rim, zygomatic arch, and frontozygomatic arch or on the lateral wall of the maxillary sinus. Significant swelling and ecchymosis are usually noted over the involved cheek and eye. Hypesthesia of the cheek is often present secondary to trauma to the infraorbital nerve at the orbital floor or rim. The facial asymmetry that occurs as a result of inward displacement of the malar eminence may be masked by edema over the fracture area. Often a stepoff may be palpated at the orbital rim and occasionally in the area of the frontozygomatic suture. Diplopia can be present as result of entrapment of orbital contents in a fracture that extends into the orbital floor. Radiographs are useful in detecting the fracture sites and the degree of displacement of the malar bone. If entrapment of orbital tissue or asymmetry of the facial bones is present, reduction of these fractures, along with repair of any defect in the orbital floor, must be performed by the otolaryngologist within five to seven days of the injury.

More severe fractures of the mid-face can occur as a result of high-velocity injuries, usually related to vehicular (automobile, bicycle) accidents. *Lefort fractures* comprise a group of mid-face fractures that present with a depressed mid-face and malocclusion. These fractures can extend into the orbits and cranial cavity. Mobility of the maxilla with stabilization of the forehead is pathognomonic of a Lefort fracture. Severe hemorrhage can accompany these fractures and may require nasal or pharyngeal packing. Cooperation among otolaryngologist, ophthalmologist, oral surgeon, and neurosurgeon is mandatory for proper treatment of these patients. Tracheotomy may be indicated if the hemorrhage or edema of the facial structures compromise the airway. Cerebrospinal fluid rhinorrhea may occur as a result of a fracture that extends through the cribriform plate. The patient is placed on bed rest with the head elevated to help decrease drainage of the cerebrospinal fluid. Antimicrobial agents are usually administered to prevent the complication of meningitis. Reduction and fixation of fractures if performed by the otolaryngologist only after other serious concomitant injuries have been treated and the child's condition permits the use of a general anesthesia. Dental consultation should be included in the management of any fracture affecting occlusion.

Barotrauma

Normally direct and open communication between the paranasal sinuses and the nasal cavities permits prompt equalization of changes in ambient pressure. If a sinus ostia is obstructed, however, changes in ambient pressure may not be transmitted to the sinus cavity, and barotrauma can result. The maxillary sinus is the sinus most commonly affected by this condition. As the child descends in an airplane (or in an underwater dive), the increased ambient pressure is transmitted to the cardiovascular system and thus to the vessels of the mucosal lining of the sinus. The mucosa becomes edematous and the vessels engorged. If the sinus is obstructed and has not equalized the air pressure, a large differential in pressure occurs between the sinus mucosa and its air-filled cavity. This results in rupture of the vessels within the mucosa and resultant bleeding into the sinus. The child will usually complain of cheek or facial pain and may have epistaxis of sinus origin. Treatment of this condition involves the use of antimicrobials (to prevent infection of the blood-filled sinus), decongestant-antihistamine therapy, and topical nasal steroids to restore the normal physiologic communication between the sinus and the nasal cavities, and avoidance of further barotrauma. The rare case that does not respond to this regimen may require referral to an otolaryngologist for further evaluation and possible sinus drainage.

Foreign Bodies

Foreign bodies in the nasal tract are common in children. Most cases present to the primary physician with a history of placing an object into the nose. In other cases, the presence of a foreign body is unsuspected and may not be discovered until the child is evaluated for a persistent, unilateral, foul-smelling, purulent rhinorrhea. Radiopaque foreign bodies, such as toys and beads, may be seen on routine sinus radiographs, but most are radiolucent, such as paper, cloth, and pieces of food. The diagnosis is made upon anterior rhinoscopy. If the object is located in the nasal vestibule, the primary physician may attempt to remove it. The foreign body can usually be removed with a small hook, forceps, or suction tip. Hygroscopic foreign bodies (such as beans), however, may swell with nasal secretions and become very difficult to remove. The foreign body should never be pushed or irrigated into the nasopharynx, where it can be aspirated by a struggling child. An otolaryngologist should be consulted if the foreign body cannot be removed easily. A general anesthetic may become necessary for the safe removal of large impacted objects. Antimicrobial agents are usually administered to prevent infection in this already traumatized area.

SUGGESTED READINGS

Bluestone C, Wald ER, Shapiro GG, et al: The diagnosis and management of sinusitis in children: Proceedings of a closed conference. *Pediatr Infect Dis* 4(6 Suppl):S61:64, 1985.

Doty R: A review of olfactory dysfunction in man. *Am J Otolaryngol* 1:57-59, 1979.

Garfinkle TS, Handler SD: Hemangiomas of the head and neck in children: Guide to management. *J Otolaryngol* 9:439-450, 1980.

Handler SD: Diagnosis and management of maxillo-facial injuries, In: Torg J (ed): Athletic Injuries to the Head, Neck and Face. Philadelphia, Lea & Febiger, 1982. pp. 223-244.

Handler SD, Raney RB: Management of neoplasms of the head and neck in children. I. Benign tumors. *Head Neck Surg* 3:395-405, 1981.

Healy GB: Approach to the nasal septum in children. *Laryngoscope* 96:1239-1242, 1986.

Jackson IT, Munro IR, Salyer KE, et al: Atlas of Craniofacial Surgery. St. Louis,   Mosby, 1982. pp. 217-257.

Refro BL: Pediatric otolaryngic allergy. *Otolaryngol Clin North Am* 25:181-196, 1992.

Rubinstein J, Handler SD: Orbital and periorbital cellulitis in children. *Head Neck Surg* 5:15-21, 1982.

Schwartz ML, Savetsky L: Choanal atresia: Clinical features, surgical approach, and long-term follow-up. *Laryngoscope* 96:1335-1339, 1986.

Sessions RB: Nasal hemorrhage. *Otolaryngol Clin North Am* 6:727-744, 1973.

Tom LWC, Anderson GJ, Womer R, et al: Nasopharyngeal malignancies in children. *Laryngoscope* 102:509-514, 1992.

Wald ER, Chiponis D, Ledesma-Medina J: Comparative effectiveness of amoxicillin and amoxicillin clavulanate potassium in acute paranasal sinus infections in children: A double-blind, placebo-controlled trial. *Pediatrics* 77:795-800, 1986.

CHAPTER 3

ORAL CAVITY AND PHARYNX

ANATOMY

The pharynx is divided into three anatomic areas: the nasopharynx, oropharynx, and hypopharynx. The cervical vertebrae form the posterior boundary of the entire pharynx. The nasopharynx is located above the soft palate, bounded anteriorly by the choanae. The oropharynx extends from the soft palate to the level of the hyoid bone. Its anterior boundary is the anterior tonsillar pillar. The hypopharynx extends from the hyoid to the esophageal inlet and surrounds the upper portion of the larynx, which is its anterior boundary (Fig 3-1).

The pharynx is partially surrounded by a muscular sheath consisting of the superior, middle, and inferior pharyngeal constrictors and the stylopharyngeus muscle. These muscles participate in the pharyngeal actions of respiration, deglutition, and phonation. The pharynx is covered by nonkeratinizing squamous epithelium throughout except for the more anterior portions of the nasopharynx, which are covered by ciliated columnar epithelium.

The oral cavity is lined with nonkeratinizing stratified squamous epithelium and contains specialized structures to assist in the processes of eating and phonation. The oral cavity also contains the teeth; the stage of develop-

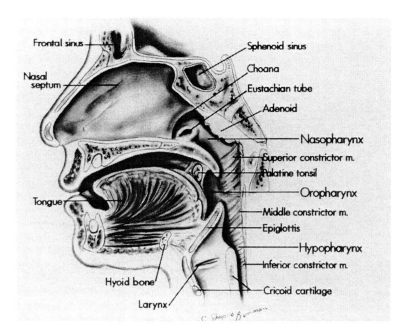

Figure 3–1. Sagittal view of pharynx, nasopharynx, oropharynx, and surrounding structures. (From Potsic WP, Handler SD, Wetmore RF: Ear, Nose, Throat and Mouth. In: Rudolph A (ed). Pediatrics. 19th ed. Norwalk, CT, Appleton & Lange, 1991.)

ment and exfoliation depends upon the age of the child. The teeth are anchored to the bone of the alveolar ridges by thick connective tissue (periodontal membrane). The primary deciduous teeth are replaced by the secondary, or permanent, teeth starting at six years of age. When fully erupted, there are 16 upper and 16 lower teeth. The two parotid ducts (Stenson's) empty on the inner surface of each cheek near the second maxillary molar. The submandibular ducts (Wharton's) are easily seen as two raised nodules on either side of the lingual frenulum. The sublingual glands empty through multiple small, poorly visible ducts along the course of the submandibular duct. Thousands of minor salivary glands are present in the submucosa of the oral cavity and pharynx.

The eustachian tube is a specialized structure that ventilates the middle ear and transports secretions from the middle ear into the nasopharynx. The medial opening of the eustachian tube lies in the anterior-inferior part of the lateral wall of the nasopharynx. The eustachian tube is cartilaginous in its medial (nasal) portion and bony in its lateral extent. The tensor veli palatini and the levator veli palatini extend from the soft palate to the orifice of the eustachian tube and assist in opening the tube during swallowing.

The blood supply to the oral cavity and pharynx is derived from branches of the external carotid artery. Its extensive vascular anastamoses provide the oral cavity and pharynx with a rich blood supply.

Sensation in the oral cavity is supplied through the fifth cranial nerve. Taste on the anterior two thirds and posterior one third of the tongue is carried by the seventh and ninth cranial nerves, respectively. The pharyngeal plexus, derived from the ninth and tenth nerves, supplied sensation to the pharynx. Motor innervation of the tongue is from the twelfth nerve. The tensor veli palatini, the main muscle controlling function of the eustachian tube, is innervated by the fifth nerve.

The oral cavity and pharynx contain the lymphoid tissue comprising Waldeyer's ring. The lingual tonsils are aggregates of lymphoid tissue on the dorsum of the posterior one third of the tongue. They merge superiorly with the palatine tonsils lying on the lateral surface of the oropharynx between the anterior and posterior tonsillar pillars. The adenoid is a mass of lymph tissue above the palate and on the superior and posterior wall of the nasopharynx. On the posterior surface of the oropharynx, small aggregates or nodules of lymphoid tissue may be present.

PHYSIOLOGY

Respiration

The oral cavity and pharynx act as a conduit for respiration in the child. The high position of the larynx and the opposition of the epiglottis to the soft palate force the neonate to breathe through the nose and nasopharynx. The oral cavity is effectively sealed off from the airway, thereby permitting simultaneous breathing and suckling. As the infant grows and the larynx descends, comfortable oral breathing is accomplished.

Alimentation

The oral cavity and pharynx also act as a conduit for the entrance of food into the body. Food entering the mouth is chewed and ground into small pieces by the action of the teeth. Salivary enzymes moisten the ingested material and start the digestive process. Deglutition begins as the tongue propels the bolus of food into the oropharynx. When this occurs, the soft palate elevates and extends posteriorly. Thus, the nasopharynx is sealed off from the oropharynx, preventing regurgitation of food into the nasal cavity. As the pharyngeal constrictor muscles propel food past the relaxed cricopharyngeal muscle (the entrance of the esophagus), the larynx elevates and the epiglottis folds posteriorly to deflect the food away from the airway. The true cords close to seal the laryngeal inlet and prevent aspiration. Neuromuscular dysfunction or delayed development may affect any stage of this process, causing nasal regurgitation, dysphagia, or aspiration.

The gag reflex is a complex neural reflex that protects against swallowing large or unpalatable objects. Reflex contractions of the pharyngeal constrictors expel foreign bodies or large boluses of food back into the oral cavity. The reflex can be modified by emotional states and can even be activated voluntarily.

Phonation

The oral cavity and pharynx are necessary for the production of intelligible speech. While the larynx creates sounds, the pharynx and oral cavity shape them into articulate speech. The tongue is the primary organ or articulation in the oral cavity; in order to produce normal speech, the tongue must be able to contact the anterior teeth and palate. The letters *m* and *n* require the passage of air into the nasopharynx and through the nose, but plosive sounds *(p, t, k)* require that the palate seal off the nasopharynx. Palatal dysfunction or nasopharyngeal obstruction can cause hypernasal or hyponasal speech, respectively.

METHODS OF EXAMINATION

Direct and Indirect Examination

Examination of the oral cavity and oropharynx is carried out by direct visualization. The structures of the oral cavity and oropharynx can be easily visualized using a bright light and a tongue blade in the patient's open mouth. The tongue blade should be placed on the anterior two thirds of the tongue in order to avoid gagging; the tongue is thereby displaced both anteriorly and inferiorly providing clear visualization of important structures. A general assessment of oral hygiene can be made by examination of the teeth and gingiva. The salivary ducts and tonsils are also visualized directly. Tongue mobility can then be assessed by asking the child to stick out or wiggle his tongue. Palatal and pharyngeal function can be noted by observing the palate and lateral pharyngeal walls when the child says "ah" or gags.

Examination of the nasopharynx and hypopharynx is most often done by indirect visualization. A small hypopharynx is most often done by indirect visualization. A small mirror held behind the palate with the tongue deflected downward will permit visualization of the nasopharynx and hypopharynx in most children over the age of three. Telescopic visualization is possible with rigid or flexible fiberoptic instruments that permit a clear view of the nasopharynx; if aimed inferiorly, the hypopharynx and larynx can be seen as well. If the child cannot cooperate for either an indirect mirror examination or telescopic visualization, an evaluation may need to be performed under general anesthesia by an otolaryngologist.

Radiologic Examination

Since the oral cavity, its contents, and surrounding structures (the salivary glands) are usually visible and easily palpated, radiographic techniques are seldom required in their evaluation. However, a lateral neck radiograph permits evaluation of the base of the tongue and the pharynx. While xeroradiography provides excellent soft tissue detail of the neck, it is rarely utilized today because of the higher radiation dose necessary to perform the study. Special views of the mandible, teeth, and salivary glands may be required in the evaluation of a process involving or affecting the oral cavity. Radioisotope scanning with ^{131}I is useful to confirm a suspected lingual thyroid. Contract cineradiography may outline masses or foreign bodies and can be used to assess the oropharyngeal phases of deglutition. Cineradiography during phonation provides the most accurate assessment of velopharyngeal function. CT and MR have become the radiologic studies of choice for any complicated abnormalities of the pharynx. CT provides excellent detail of bone-tissue interfaces, while MR is superior for soft tissue detail.

COMMON COMPLAINTS

Sore Throat

Sore throat is a symptom common to many disorders of the pharynx and larynx. The sensation of throat pain is conveyed to the brain by way of efferent fibers from the glossopharyngeal nerve and the internal division of the superior laryngeal nerve. The most common cause of pain in the throat is the *viral upper respiratory infection*. While an upper respiratory infection is most often generalized to the entire upper respiratory system (nose, paranasal sinuses, pharynx, and larynx), pharyngeal and laryngeal involvement is responsible for the feeling of a sore throat. The patient will often complain of malaise, a sore, scratchy throat, and pain on swallowing (odynophagia). Physical examination of the child will indicate the signs of pharyngeal infection: fever, erythematous pharyngeal mucosa, tonsillar exudate (if tonsils are present), and tender cervical adenopathy. Indirect laryngoscopy will reveal erythematous, supraglottic (arytenoids and aryepiglottic folds) and glottic (vocal cords) structures.

Other inflammatory sources of pharyngeal/laryngeal irritation, such as *infectious mononucleosis, herpangina, aphthous ulceration*, and *bacterial pharyngitis/tonsillitis*, may cause a sore throat. Treatment of the sore throat caused by any of these infections will depend on the responsible agent. Soft diet, antipyretics, voice rest, topical and systemic analgesics and antimicrobial agents, when appropriate, are useful adjuvants in the treatment of these processes.

Other infections involving the larynx, such as *croup* and *epiglottitis*, can present with a sore throat. However, since the associated symptoms of respiratory distress and stridor are often severe, the appropriate diagnostic and therapeutic strategies are directed toward the respiratory distress rather than toward the sore throat.

Breathing air of *low humidity* has a drying effect on the respiratory epithelium, injuring the ciliated cells and altering the mucociliary transport system of the respiratory tract. Mild pharyngeal irritation results, producing a sore throat. The dried surface cells are also more susceptible to infection.

The possibility of *local inhaled irritants* as the cause of a sore throat should be explored with the parent or caretaker. For example, an adolescent who smokes cigarettes or a child living with parents who smoke may complain of a chronic sore throat. Marihuana smoke is particularly irritating to the pharynx. The smoke is often hot and may even cause a first-degree burn of the mucosa. Rebreathing the smoke prolongs its contact with the pharyngeal surface. Often overlooked as a cause of sore throat is the smoke that leaks into the house from a fireplace. An early evening fire can be a source of pharyngeal irritation all night. Hobby and craft materials may contain *dusts* and *hydrocarbons* (e.g., from glues or solvents) that can also cause a sore throat.

An *allergic diathesis* is another factor responsible for a chronic sore throat. Seasonal or perennial allergy results in an increased and thickened mucus secretion, making the child aware of a postnasal drip and a sense of throat irritation.

Other causes of sore throat include *trauma, cricoarytenoid arthritis* (related to juvenile rheumatoid arthritis), *foreign body* and *neoplasm*. These possibilities must be considered in the evaluation of a child with an atypical sore throat or one that fails to respond to conventional treatment. A history of trauma or of possible foreign body ingestion should alert the primary physician to the possible etiology of the sore throat. Lateral neck radiographs may be helpful in demonstrating the presence of a foreign body, retropharyngeal air (indicating pharyngeal perforation or infection), or a mass lesion. An otolaryngologist should be consulted in the evaluation of a child presenting with an unusual or atypical sore throat. Occasionally, direct laryngoscopy may be necessary to determine the etiology of the sore throat in order to institute appropriate therapy. While small pharyngeal lacerations will usually heal spontaneously, larger tears will require primary repair and possible exploration of the neck. Removal of a foreign body requires endoscopy under a general anesthetic. If a suspicious lesion is found in the larynx of a child complaining of an atypical sore throat, a biopsy should be obtained.

Drooling

Drooling may be caused by increased production of saliva, an inability (voluntary or involuntary) to swallow saliva, or a combination of both. Since the production of saliva is influenced by both neural and local factors, several conditions may contribute to a relative overproduction of salivary fluids. *Local factors* that can cause increased salivary flow include stomatitis, chewing, erupting primary teeth, mucous membrane irritants (e.g., spices such as pepper), cigarette smoke, peppermint, and quinine. Neurally mediated factors are conducted through the autonomic nervous system; they include drugs (parasympathomimetics, sympatholytics), heavy metal poisoning, and rabies.

Drooling may also be caused by the child's *inability or unwillingness to swallow a normal amount of saliva*. This may be caused by any lesion which blocks the passage of saliva from the mouth to the esophagus. Tonsillar enlargement, foreign bodies, neoplasms and esophageal stenosis can all impede the movement of saliva. In fact, drooling and unwillingness to swallow saliva may be the only sign of an esophageal foreign body ingestion. A child may decide, voluntarily or involuntarily, not to initiate swallowing because of psychological factors or pain related to oral or pharyngeal trauma (e.g., post-tonsillectomy), infections (such as tonsillitis, peritonsillar abscess or epiglottitis), or caustic ingestion.

Because swallowing is a complex action, anything that interferes with *neuromuscular function* can lead to uncoordinated swallowing attempts and drooling. Infants drool frequently partly because of their immature nervous systems. Children with neuromuscular disorders will drool for the same reason. Resolution of this symptom will depend on the developmental progress and potential of the child.

Management of drooling requires a complete history and otolaryngologic examination with appropriate radiographs as indicated. If a cause for the symptom is found, appropriate treatment should be instituted. If the drooling persists or no obvious cause is detected, the child should be referred to an otolaryngologist for evaluation and treatment.

CONGENITAL MALFORMATIONS

Congenital malformations of the oral cavity and pharynx are relatively common. While many are of little clinical significance, others such as a cleft palate deformity have serious potential problems and require long-term care. A common abnormality is a short lingual frenulum (*ankyloglossia*) or *tongue-tie*. This entity is of little significance unless tongue mobility is restricted severely enough to cause problems with speech, eating, or recurrent trauma to the tongue and frenulum from the teeth. Mild to moderate ankyloglossia causes no difficulty with eating, speech, or dental development. Referral of these patients, to an otolaryngologist may be helpful to reassure the family that, in most cases, nothing needs to be done and no functional deficit will develop. Release of a severe and clinically significant tongue-tie can be performed if any dysfunction becomes apparent.

The shape of the oral cavity may be altered by branchial arch and stomodeum developmental anomalies. *Macrostomia* or *microstomia* may occur and are usually only of cosmetic significance. Small oral structure and intraoral asymmetry may be associated with unilateral defects in *mandibular development*. These may become both cosmetically and functionally important as the child grows and teeth develop.

The most common oropharyngeal malformations occur in the palate. A *high-arched palate* is probably a normal anatomic variant and is only significant in that it decreases the size of the nasal cavity and nasopharynx and may predispose these children to nasal and nasopharyngeal obstruction and/or infections. *Congenital short palate, palatal paresis*, or *paralysis* can all cause velopharyngeal incompetence and hypernasal speech.

A bifid uvula, while of no clinical significance in itself, may indicate the presence of a more important submucous cleft palate. In a *submucous cleft palate*, there is incomplete fusion of the muscles in the midline of the soft palate. Usually there is a translucent bluish-appearing area in the midline of the soft palate where the palatal aponeurosis is absent. Often, a notch in the posterior edge of the bone of the hard palate can be palpated where it joins the soft palate. Submucous cleft palates are of clinical significance only if they are associated with velopharyngeal incompetence or recurrent ear disease. Since the palatal closure in a child with a submucous cleft palate is weaker than in a normal child, a child with a submucous cleft palate and normal speech may develop velopharyngeal incompetence if an adenoidectomy is done. *Cleft palate deformity* may occur alone or in association with a cleft lip. These patients often require feeding with a special long nipple to facilitate sucking and entrance of food into the pharynx without causing nasal regurgitation. Surgical repair of the lip and palate is deferred until the child is approximately three months and one year old, respectively. Since almost all patients with a cleft palate deformity have secretory otitis media as well, they should be referred to an otolaryngologist for management of this chronic disorder.

Cysts may occur anywhere in the oral cavity and pharynx. Small to moderate size *mucoceles* (mucous-membrane lined cysts) may occur at any place in the oral cavity where minor salivary glands are present. These mucoceles often will break spontaneously and may not recur. However, if they recur after spontaneous drainage or simple incision and drainage, excision is required. *Epithelial inclusion* cysts also occur in the oral cavity and are most commonly seen at lines of embryonic fusion such as the midline of the tongue or palate. While they also may break and drain spontaneously, excision is usually required. A *ranula* is a large cystic dilation of one of the sublingual glands lying along the submandibular duct. The cyst presents under the tongue and may cause dysphagia, airway obstruction, or both. Marsupialization (exteriorization) or complete excision of the cyst, preserving the submandibular duct, is required to prevent recurrence. A cystic mass may occur at the base of the tongue when the thyroid fails to descent into the neck and remains in the oral cavity as a *lingual thyroid*. A radioisotope (^{131}I) scan will confirm whether this mass is thyroid tissue. A child with a lingual thyroid does not require surgical removal of the mass unless it is extremely large and interferes with respiration or deglutition. Lingual thyroid tissue tends to become hypoactive as the years pass, so these patients should have occasional thyroid function tests to determine when, and if, thyroid replacement becomes necessary.

Congenital pharyngeal masses include *encephaloceles, teratomas, dermoids, Tornwaldt's cyst* (persistent cystic remnant of the notochord), and *branchial pouch remnants. Pharyngeal stenosis* and *webs* are rare but may cause severe respiratory distress in the neonate. *Congenital absence of the pharyngeal tonsils* may indicate a generalized immune deficiency state such as *Di George syndrome (thymic aplasia)* or *X-linked agammaglobulinemia.* An *eruption cyst* is a bluish mass that often appears on the alveolus just before a primary tooth is about to erupt. These cysts cause no difficulty and require no treatment.

The assistance of an otolaryngologist can be quite helpful in the management of patients with congenital deformities of the mouth or pharynx. Often a simple-appearing mass will have far-reaching implications and will require special expertise for proper treatment.

INFECTIOUS DISEASES

Viral Infections

Aphthous ulcers are painful buccal, lingual, or pharyngeal ulcers that recur from time to time. The precise etiology of aphthous ulcerations is unknown but is thought to be viral. No specific therapy is helpful, and the ulcers resolve in seven to ten days without treatment. Particularly large or painful ulcers can be treated with Mile's mixture, a combination of liquid tetracycline, hydrocortisone, and viscous lidocaine in Orabase®. *Herpes simplex virus* usually causes recurrent bouts of isolated lip eruptions, but primary Herpes simplex stomatitis is associated with a viral syndrome of fever and malaise for one to two days prior to vesicle eruption and subsequent ulcer formation. Usually, severe gingivitis is evident, but the pharynx is relatively spared of ulcerations. The ulcers heal in seven to ten days without specific treatment. *Herpangina (Coxsackie A)* infections causes severe ulcerative pharyngitis. Initially, discrete vesicles appear, which then rupture to form ulcers. Herpangina usually affects the pharynx and posterior oral cavity, tending to spare the anterior mouth. The infection tends to be epidemic and begins to resolve without treatment in seven to ten days. Supportive therapy with viscous lidocaine mouthwash (to permit eating), systemic analgesics and adequate fluid intake is helpful until the painful viral lesions that occur in the above syndromes resolve.

Herpes zoster oticus is a varicella-zoster viral infection that presents with unilateral vesicular ear eruption, facial nerve paralysis, sensorineural hearing loss, and oropharyngeal ulcers. The mouth ulcers usually occur in the oropharyngeal distribution of the ninth cranial (glossopharyngeal) nerve. Severe vertigo may also occur in this condition. While the ulcers resolve with disappearance of the zoster eruption, postherpetic pharyngeal or otitic neuralgia may persist.

Measles usually presents with signs of a mild upper respiratory infection. Koplik's spots appear a few days before the skin rash and are white or bluish spots surrounded by an area of erythema on the inside of the cheek near the opening of the parotid duct. *Chicken pox (varicella)* vesicles may also occur in the oral and pharyngeal mucosa. The vesicles rupture to form white or gray ulcers that disappear when the skin lesions begin to form a crust.

The most common viral pharyngeal infection is an *acute viral pharyngitis*. Since this pharyngitis is often one component of the common cold or upper respiratory infection, the responsible agents include *adenovirus, rhinovirus, coronavirus*, and *parainfluenzae*. The pharyngitis is rarely an isolated inflammatory process and is usually associated with tonsillitis (if tonsils are present), rhinitis, sinusitis, and less frequently laryngitis, tracheitis and bronchitis. The pharynx is erythematous, and an exudate may be present. Fever, malaise, and tender cervical adenopathy are usually present. Culture of the pharyngeal mucosa is the only way to differentiate a viral from a bacterial pharyngeal infection. Treatment for a viral pharyngitis is symptomatic, with fluids and antipyretics/analgesics. Antibiotics are of little use except to prevent secondary bacterial infection. During an acute viral upper respiratory infection, the host defenses in the upper respiratory tract are altered; acute suppurative otitis media, bacterial sinusitis, or suppurative cervical adenitis may develop in children.

Infectious mononucleosis is a generalized viral syndrome caused by *Epstein-Barr virus,* which presents with fever, malaise, pharyngitis, and generalized tender enlarged lymphadenopathy. While the clinical picture, with appropriate blood tests, will lead to the correct diagnosis of infectious mononucleosis, the appearance of the pharynx itself is nonspecific. The tonsils are generally markedly enlarged, with a whitish exudate over the surface. Occasionally, *Streptococcus* is cultured from the tonsillar surface. Dysphagia and/or airway obstruction are seen in varying degrees depending upon the severity of the infection. Treatment is supportive; most cases have an uneventful recovery. The use of amoxicillin or ampicillin in children with infectious mononucleosis should be avoided due to a high incidence of rashes. The enlarged lymph nodes of infectious mononucleosis respond dramatically to corticosteroids, but their use should be restricted to cases of significant airway obstruction. Those children with either hematologic or airway complications of infectious mononucleosis require hospitalization for further evaluation and treatment. If medical management of infectious mononucleosis fails to relieve airway obstruction, intervention with a nasopharyngeal airway or intubation may be required.

Bacterial Infections

Bacterial infection in the oral cavity is most often a result of the combination of a *nonsyphilitic spirochete* and *Fusobacterium.* The interaction of these two agents causes acute *necrotizing ulcerative gingivitis*, or *trenchmouth.* The infection usually occurs in cases of poor oral hygiene and is not communicable. Presenting symptoms include the sudden onset of severe pain, drooling, and bleeding gums. There is a foul odor to the breath, and the dental papillae and gingival margins are often ulcerated. Uncomplicated trenchmouth should be treated by local debridement and vigorous brushing of the teeth and gums with a soft toothbrush. This process is often quite painful and may be accompanied by bleeding gums. Hydrogen peroxide (2%) in water as a mouthwash three times per day will also help improve oral hygiene. Antibiotics (penicillin) may be beneficial in severe or persistent cases.

A spirochete-fusobacterial infection that spreads to the tonsillar and posterior pharyngeal area is called *Vincent's angina.* Nutritional support, hydration, and high-dose intravenous antibiotic (penicillin) therapy should be used in conjunction with local oral treatment. Fulminant infection may also cause necrosis of the cheek and lips (cancrum oris) as well.

Most often, bacterial infections of the pharynx occur as simple infectious processed caused by organisms such as *Group A ß-hemolytic Streptococcus, Streptococcus pneumoniae, Hemophilius influenzae*, and *Staphylococcus aureus.* However, some authorities believe that the bacterial component may represent proliferation of these organisms during an acute viral upper respiratory infection, and not a primary infection.

Acute bacterial pharyngitis presents in a fashion similar to that seen in an acute viral pharyngitis, but differentiation between these two entities can only be made with a throat culture. Pharyngitis is too restrictive a term because the process usually affects not only the pharyngeal wall, but the contents of the pharynx (i.e., the tonsils and adenoids) as well. While in any one child, during any one illness, one area of the pharynx may appear to be more affected by the inflammatory process, the infection is more correctly termed *pharyngotonsillitis* or *adenotonsillitis*, indicating its generalized nature. The component contributed by pharyngitis consists of erythematous and swollen lateral and posterior pharyngeal walls. Tonsillitis is noted by swollen, erythematous tonsils with a whitish exudate over the surface. Nasal congestion and purulent nasal or postnasal discharge are frequent signs of adenoiditis. Fever, malaise, and cervical adenitis frequently accompany these bouts of pharyngotonsillitis. Treatment consists of a 10-day course of antibiotics (usually penicillin or amoxicillin) after appropriate cultures have been taken.

When pharyngotonsillitis extends to the peritonsillar tissues, *peritonsillar cellulitis* or *abscess* may occur. In the former, the tonsil bulges forward and medially and appears much larger than the opposite tonsil. The anterior tonsillar pillar on that side is usually acutely inflamed. Peritonsillar cellulitis causes a sore throat that is most severe on the affected side but does not often cause trismus. Treatment requires high-dose intravenous antibiotics (penicillin or cephalosporin). When the cellulitis progresses, purulent material collects in the space between the tonsillar capsule and the parapharyngeal muscles, forming a peritonsillar abscess. This presents with further medial and forward displacement of the involved tonsil, swelling and bulging of the soft palate and anterior tonsillar pillar, severe pain, "hot potato" voice, and trismus. Peritonsillar abscess will usually resolve if treated with intravenous antibiotics (penicillin, cephalosporin or clindamycin) for seven to ten days. However, needle aspiration, formal incision and drainage, or immediate tonsillectomy (which also accomplishes complete drainage) hasten recovery and decrease the hospital stay. If an acute tonsillectomy is not performed, most otolaryngologists recommend a tonsillectomy six weeks later to prevent recurrence of the peritonsillar abscess.

Pharyngotonsillitis may cause suppurative adenitis of the retropharyngeal or parapharyngeal lymph nodes, leading to the development of a *retropharyngeal* or *parapharyngeal abscess*, respectively. These abscesses can extend in the tissue planes (of the neck) from the base of the skull to the mediastinum. Airway obstruction from mechanical obstruction or laryngeal edema as well as aspiration of purulent material from spontaneous drainage of the abscess make these complications of pharyngotonsillitis potentially lethal. A retropharyngeal abscess is usually well demonstrated on a lateral neck radiography (Fig. 3-2), while a parapharyngeal abscess causes dramatic lateral pharyngeal fullness and neck swelling. Treatment consists of hospitalization, intravenous antibiotics, and prompt surgical drainage of the abscess.

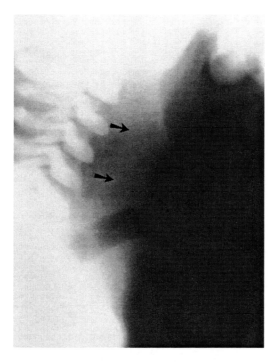

Figure 3–2. Radiograph demonstrating retropharyngeal abcess. Air in soft tissues is from gas-producing organisms. Note widened retropharyngeal space (arrows).

The management of recurrent bacterial adenotonsillitis has been a matter of controversy for many years. The merits of medical management versus surgical intervention have been debated without resolution. Proponents of medical therapy point to the anesthetic risk and operative mortality to justify their position. Conversely, while long-term or prophylactic courses of penicillin may be helpful in reducing the frequency of streptococcal pharyngitis, the use of antibiotics is not without risk of the development of an allergic reaction or secondary resistant infection. Tonsillectomy and adenoidectomy decrease the frequency of adenotonsillitis and pharyngitis. While some authorities have claimed that removal of the tonsils and adenoids may result in decreased immunity to infections, no such decrease in the local or systemic immune response has ever been documented. Since there is no clear, widely accepted mode of treatment at this time, management must be individualized for each child. The frequency and severity of the bouts of pharyngotonsillitis together with the child's morbidity (school missed, days bedridden, history of cardiac disease, antibiotic reactions, upper airway obstruction, risk of anesthesia) and various social parameters (work missed by parents, siblings exposed to infectious process) must be taken into account when deciding upon medical versus surgical management.

Diphtheria is a rare cause of pharyngotonsillitis but still occurs sporadically. It presents with a thick grayish membrane over the surface of the pharynx that causes bleeding if it is removed. If the membrane extends to the larynx or trachea, airway obstruction may result. Humidification, intravenous antibiotic therapy, and the removal of any obstructing membrane are the mainstays of therapy.

Gonococcal pharyngitis is being encountered more frequently in the adolescent age group. It has no distinguishing features and can only be differentiated from viral or other bacterial pharyngitis by Gram stain and culture. High-dose intramuscular antibiotic therapy (usually penicillin) is the appropriate treatment. The increasing incidence of penicillin-resistant gonococci makes these infections difficult to treat; culture and sensitivity tests are crucial to management of these cases.

Actinomyocosis sulfur granules are normally found in the crypts of tonsils, but a clinically apparent oropharyngeal actinomyocosis infection occurs rarely. It usually follows a puncture of the oral mucosa by a foreign body. The infection is characterized by an ulcerated oral lesion with a draining sinus tract to the submandibular region. Cervical adenopathy is common. Treatment requires high-dose long-term penicillin therapy and excision of all infected tissue including sinus tracts.

Fungal Infections

Fungal infections of the oral cavity and pharynx usually occur in nutritionally debilitated or immunosuppressed patients or in those who have altered oropharyngeal flora from antibiotic therapy. The most frequent fungal infection is *candidiasis (thrush)*. Oropharyngeal *Candida* infection appears as white patches adherent to the underlying mucosa with surrounding erythema; although the mucosa may appear diffusely inflamed with the white patches being small and relatively inconspicuous. Oropharyngeal *Candida* is treated with oral nystatin and correction of any underlying predisposing factors. Yogurt may be eaten to reestablish normal oral flora and to create an acid environment in the oropharynx in order to hinder further bacterial or fungal overgrowth.

Mucormycosis can present as a fulminating infection of the nasal, sinus, and periorbital tissues. It usually occurs in young, poorly controlled insulin-dependent diabetics who are in ketoacidosis. Its presentation in the oral cavity and pharynx is noted by a black eschar of the soft or hard palate. The fungal elements cause thrombosis of small blood vessels, leading to painless necrosis of the affected tissue. The ophthalmic complications are severe, resulting in ophthalmoplegia and blindness. Fulminant infections may become rapidly fatal with intracranial spread. Treatment requires systemic amphotericin B and surgical debridement of necrotic tissue.

ALLERGIC AND NONINFECTIOUS CONDITIONS

Allergic diatheses may affect the oral cavity or pharynx alone, but most often the involvement of these structures is only part of a more generalized allergic response. In the oral cavity, migrating patches of desquamation on the tongue (*geographic tongue*) are thought to be of allergic origin. Similarly, prominent *lymphoid nodules* on the posterior pharyngeal wall are thought to be atopy related. Treatment of these entities is symptomatic, with attention to any underlying allergic cause.

Oropharyngeal inflammation and ulceration may occur from noninfectious causes, of which *erythema multiforme* (*Stevens-Johnson syndrome*) is the most dramatic. It occurs in children and young adults and is characterized by fever, papular skin lesions, and mucous membrane bullae. The skin vesicles rupture to form large confluent ulcerations that bleed easily and form large areas of crusts. Erythema multiforme is thought to be an allergic phenomenon usually associated with recent use of a sulfa drug, penicillin, cefaclor or barbituate. Treatment consists of hospitalization and hydration. Use of systemic steroids is controversial. The drug initiating the disease should be stopped immediately. Antibiotics are employed only if secondary infection occurs.

A rare condition that may cause disturbingly large oral and pharyngeal ulceration is *necrotizing sialometaplasia*. This benign inflammatory process of the minor salivary glands usually heals slowly over several weeks, regardless of treatment. Biopsy is usually required to rule out an underlying malignancy.

Another noninfectious intraoral problem occasionally seen in children and young adults is *gingival hyperplasia*. This condition occurs during periods of hormonal changes (such as puberty, pregnancy, or the use of birth control pills) or therapy with phenytoin sodium (Dilantin). Good intraoral hygiene, restoration of normal hormonal balance, and discontinuance of any possible causative drug may help prevent and relieve gingival hyperplasia.

LYMPHOID HYPERPLASIA

Hyperplasia of the lymphoid tissue of the pharynx, especially the tonsils and adenoids, is a common condition in children. Although the actual etiology of this lymphoid enlargement is unknown, allergy and chronic or recurrent infection seem to be the most likely causes.

Marked enlargement of the tonsils and adenoids may cause chronic upper airway obstruction and, subsequently, many significant problems. Mouth-breathing, a common symptom in children with lymphoid hyperplasia, dries the oral mucosa and alters oral flora, predisposing children to dental caries and recurrent upper respiratory tract infection. Since upward pressure by the tongue is required for proper palatal growth and alignment of the upper teeth, chronic mouth-breathing is association with a high incidence of midface hypoplasia and orthodontic problems. Speech is usually garbled and hyponasal; the child sounds as if he or she "has a cold" all the time. Weight gain may be poor secondary to eating habits affected by the decreased sense of smell and dysphagia caused by large tonsils blocking the opening to the pharynx. Altered nasopharyngeal and oropharyngeal physiology can cause eustachian tube dysfunction and resultant secretory or recurrent suppurative otitis media. Severe airway obstruction is associated with hypoxia, hypercapnea, and sleep apnea, which may lead to chronic sleep deprivation, behavioral disorders (somnolence or hyperactivity), as well as pulmonary hypertension and right heart failure (cor pulmonale).

Many children with significant airway obstruction will appear relatively normal during the day (and in the physician's office), but these same children can be severely obstructed and have prolonged periods of apnea when sleeping. While the most accurate manner of documenting sleep apnea is by monitoring the child in a specialized sleep laboratory, an effective and inexpensive way of demonstrating obstructive sleep patterns is to have the parents record an audio or video tape of the child during sleep. A lateral neck radiograph in the supine position may also be helpful in demonstrating the site of obstruction in the nasopharynx or oropharynx. Children with obstructive apnea or any of the other complications of chronic airway obstruction should be referred to an otolaryngologist for further evaluation.

NEOPLASMS

Benign Neoplasms

Benign neoplasms of many types may present in the oral cavity. The tissue of origin may be the mucosa or any of the surrounding tissues, such as teeth, bone, or the major and minor salivary glands.

Hemangiomas, lymphangiomas, teratomas, and *neurofibromas* may appear almost anywhere in the oral cavity or pharynx. In general, the treatment of these benign tumors is surgical excision. If the diagnosis is obvious, as in most cases of hemangiomas and lymphangiomas, the lesions can be observed for growth or any sign of a complication. This philosophy of observation is especially appropriate for hemangiomas that often involute after a 12 to 18 month period of growth. Treatment — including systemic steroids, laser surgery, or surgical excision — is reserved for those patients with airway obstruction, systemic hematologic or cardiovascular complications, dysphagia, severe cosmetic deformity, or for those cases in which the diagnosis is not clear. Swellings in the salivary glands or oropharynx may be *tumors of salivary gland origin.* Surgical excision is usually required in order to determine whether the mass is histologically benign. Intraparotid hemangiomas are common in children and will most often resolve spontaneously (see Chapter 5 for further details).

An uncommon but important benign neoplasm presenting in the nasopharynx is the *nasopharyngeal juvenile angiofibroma,* which occurs almost exclusively in prepubescent and adolescent males. It presents with recurrent or massive epistaxis, nasal obstruction, secretory otitis media, and hyponasal speech. Nasopharynx juvenile angiofibroma appears as a large intranasal or nasopharyngeal mass with an edematous bluish appearance. It is often confused with nasal polyps, swollen turbinates, or adenoid hypertrophy. Radiographs will often demonstrate an obstructing nasopharyngeal mass with anterior bowing of the posterior wall of the maxillary sinus. Office biopsy of these masses should be avoided, as it may result in life-threatening hemorrhage. The child should be referred to an otolaryngologist for further evaluation. Treatment includes arteriographic embolization followed by complete surgical excision. Subsequent radiation therapy may also be considered but is usually reserved for recurrent tumors or those with intracranial extension.

A lesion with a disturbing appearance that is occasionally seen in the child and adolescent is the *pyogenic granuloma* or *epulis*. There is considerable controversy regarding the precise nature of this entity — whether it is a neoplasms or an inflammatory response. It appears as an ulcerated mass that is friable and that bleeds intermittently. In young children, the undersurface of the tongue near the frenulum is a common site of occurrence. In older children, the gingiva or portion of the tongue near a recent dental restoration is a common location. Pregnancy may predispose an adolescent to the formation of a pyogenic granuloma. Since trauma, chronic irritation, and altered hormonal states (i.e., pregnancy) appear to be etiologic in the development of these lesions, correction of these factors will often help in the resolution of this pyogenic granuloma. Treatment should be directed toward removing the source of irritation. Sharp teeth can be coated and dental appliances revised. However, total excision or curettage of the lesion is usually required for a complete cure. This finding lends support to the possibility that this lesion is neoplastic in origin.

Malignant Neoplasms

Malignant neoplasms of the oral cavity are uncommon in children and adolescents. The pharynx is one of the more common sites in the head and neck region for *rhabdomyosarcomas, lymphomas,* and *squamous cell carcinomas (lymphoepitheliomas).* Nasal obstruction, epistaxis, and hyponasal speech are common presenting symptoms of these tumors. Cranial nerve palsies and prominent cervical adenopathy are all signs of advanced disease but are all too often seen at the initial examination. The histologic diagnosis is made on the basis of tumor biopsy. Treatment usually consists of a combination of radiotherapy and chemotherapy. Localized disease in the head and neck without intracranial spread or distant metastasis is usually associated with a good survival rate.

Malignant salivary gland tumors may occur within the major or minor salivary glands. The management of these tumors in children is the same as that in adults. Surgical excision, radiation therapy, and chemotherapy are required, depending on the nature and extent of the neoplasm.

Any patient with a tumor or suspected tumor in the oral cavity, pharynx, salivary glands, or neck should be referred to an otolaryngologist for a complete head and neck examination, including the nasopharynx, oropharynx, and hypopharynx. A surgical procedure (biopsy or excision) is required to establish the diagnosis and ensure correct treatment.

TRAUMA

Traumatic injuries to the oral cavity and pharynx can range from those that are trivial in nature to life-threatening emergencies. Fortunately, trauma to the oral cavity is often minor (usually self-inflicted by biting the cheek or tongue). While this is often painful and may cause hemorrhage or hematoma formation, treatment is usually unnecessary.

Lacerations of the tongue can occur when the lower jaw is hit suddenly trapping the tongue between the teeth. These lacerations, while disturbing to parent and child alike, heal without functional or cosmetic deformity unless the basic structural integrity of the tongue is disrupted. Suturing of the tongue is required only in those cases in which significant hemorrhage or a deep laceration is threatening the viability or function of a portion of the tongue. An otolaryngologist can often assist the primary practitioner in this determination.

Large *lacerations of the cheek* can occur as a result of the forceful introduction of a pointed foreign body into the mouth (such as a child falling with a stick in his or her mouth) or in association with more severe trauma such as a mandibular fracture. Again, most of these lacerations heal spontaneously without sequelae. Large buccal lacerations occurring through-and-through the cheek or through which buccal fat protrudes probably deserve careful examination (usually under a general anesthetic) to search for associated injuries (e.g., to facial nerve or parotid duct) as well as formal closure.

Lacerations of the palate and tonsils are most common when an patient falls with an object such as a pencil or stick in his mouth. While these lacerations may appear large and gaping, suture repair is rarely needed. Large wounds may require formal exploration and repair for hemostasis or to prevent the formation of a palatal fistula with subsequent hypernasal speech. The heeling of these larger lacerations may be facilitated by a course of antibiotic therapy.

Penetrating wounds of the pharynx permit contamination of the pharyngeal tissues with oral flora. This can lead to a retropharyngeal or parapharyngeal abscess. The presence of a perforation can be determined by feeling crepitation in the neck or by the appearance of air on a lateral neck radiograph. The carotid artery, jugular vein, and cranial and cervical nerves lie lateral to the pharynx and deep penetrating wounds can damage these structures. Airway protection is of paramount concern in the management of these patients. Endotracheal intubation or tracheostomy may be required to clean an obstructed airway. The patient should be referred immediately to an otolaryngologist for endoscopic evaluation and possible repair of the perforated viscous.

Minor dental trauma is probably more frequent than commonly appreciated. A chipped or even temporarily loosened tooth may not be brought to a parent's, let alone a physician's, attention. *Chipped teeth* without exposed dentin or dental pulp require no immediate treatment. These teeth can be distinguished from those that are more severely injured because they are not sensitive to change in temperature. Exposed dentin is painful, and the child may requires analgesics for pain relief. An analgesic and protective compound should be applied for pain relief and protection. If the pulp is exposed and, therefore, contaminated with oral flora, antibiotics should be given. Any child with a chipped or fractured tooth that is painful or sensitive to change in temperature should be seen by a dentist as soon as possible. Definitive dental restoration can be carried out electively.

Mildly loosened teeth often need no treatment except the institution of a soft diet to avoid further loosening and to promote refixation. Very loose teeth may benefit from a splint or arch bar to secure the loosened teeth to the adjacent stable dentition. Loose teeth may take three to four weeks to stabilize.

An *avulsed secondary tooth* should be replaced immediately in its socket. If this is not done easily, the tooth should be kept in the patient's mouth under the tongue, where the saliva will preserve the viability of the periodontal ligaments. If a young child cannot be trusted to keep the tooth under the tongue, the can tooth can be preserved by a parent by placing the tooth under his or her tongue until it can be reimplanted in the child's mouth. The tooth can also be placed in milk if the patent is offended by the idea of placing a tooth under his or her tongue. If the tooth has fallen into the dirt, it should be gently washed off with cool water and placed in the socket or under the tongue. An avulsed tooth should never be brushed or wiped off because this destroys the periodontal ligament. Deciduous teeth are not reimplanted because of the potential damage this can cause to the deeper, secondary teeth. A dentist should be consulted as soon as possible for all tooth avulsion injuries. The reimplanted tooth must be immobilized and splinted to identify retained root tips, incompletely fractured teeth, and associated mandibular fractures.

Mandibular fractures are fairly common in children and young adults and usually result from striking the chin on a hard surface. The fracture most frequently occurs in the subcondylar region. Fractures of the angle or body of the mandible often communicate with the oral cavity and present with intraoral bleeding. Pain and swelling over the lower jaw develop rapidly, and there is usually trismus as well as malocclusion. Even young children will notice that their teeth do not seem to fit.

Immediate care should be directed to protecting the airway and clearing the oral cavity of fractured teeth to prevent aspiration. A snug head dressing will support the mandible and relieve pain by reducing jaw mobility. For patients suspected of having a fractured mandible, mandibular radiographs should be obtained to define the fracture (or fractures, as is more commonly the case), followed by referral to an otolaryngologist for further management.

Caustic ingestion most often occurs accidentally in children but can be a suicidal attempt or gesture in adolescents. Caustics (alkaline or acid) may cause burns that range from mild (first degree) to full-thickness loss of pharyngeal tissue (third degree). Alkaline substances cause the most severe burns by liquidification necrosis. Acid burns are usually more limited because of their coagulation necrosis. Mild first-degree burns require no treatment, but severe burns may be associated with respiratory distress and later pharyngeal stenosis. Since the nature and extent of the burn can seldom be determined on the initial examination of the oral cavity, the child should be referred to an otolaryngologist who can perform the necessary endoscopy within 24 hours. By this time, the areas that have been burned will have become demarcated to permit proper assessment of the injury. The absence of an oral burn does not rule out serious burns further along the alimentary tract. In addition, the oropharyngeal burn may be only the beginning of an extensive life-threatening esophageal burn requiring early endoscopic diagnosis and immediate management.

FOREIGN BODIES

Foreign bodies of the oral cavity or pharynx are not common because of the protective mechanism of the tongue and pharynx (gag reflex) that expels foreign materials. However, fish bones, pins, or sharp toys can become stuck in the oral mucosa, tonsils, or pharynx (Fig. 3-3). If the object can be seen and grasped easily with forceps, it should be removed by the primary practitioner. If this cannot be done easily, or bleeding is associated with the injury, an otolaryngologist should be consulted.

Occasionally food will lodge in the hypopharynx; these pieces of food must be removed endoscopically. Large objects that are too big to pass into the esophagus may remain in the hypopharynx and cause respiratory distress. If the child is able to talk and is breathing adequately, no attempt should be made to remove the foreign body in the office. The physician

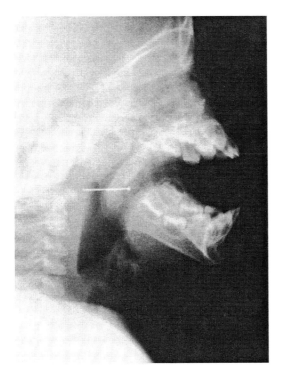

Figure 3–3. Radiograph demonstrating straight pin in the pharynx.

should not stick his fingers into the child's pharynx to attempt removal of a large object, as this may only push the object down farther and block the airway completely.

If the child with a pharyngeal foreign body is unable to breathe or phonate, a true emergency exists. Immediate intervention is required to save the child's life. The Heimlich maneuver or back slaps should be instituted in an attempt to dislodge the material from the hypopharynx and laryngeal inlet (see also Chapter 4).

SUGGESTED READINGS

Bernstein L: Dental development and abnormalities. In: Healy GB (ed): Common Problems in Pediatric Otolaryngology. Chicago, Year Book Medical Publishers, 1990. pp. 303-322.

Crysdale WS, Greenberg J, Koheil R, et al: The drooling patient: Team evaluation and management. *Int J Pediatr Otorhinolaryngol* 9:241-248, 1985.

Friedman M, Brenski A, Taylor L: Treatment of aphthous ulcers in AIDS patients. *Laryngoscope* 104:566-570, 1994.

Kaban LB. Pediatric Oral and Maxillofacial Surgery. Philadelphia, W.B. Saunders Co., 1990. pp. 161-260.

Laskaris G. Color Atlas of Oral Diseases. New York, Thieme Medical Publishers, 1988.

Paradise JL, Bluestone CD, Bachman RZ, et al: Efficacy of tonsillectomy for recurrent throat infection in severely affected children. *N Engl J Med* 310:674-683, 1984.

Potsic WP, Marsh RR: Snoring and obstructive sleep apnea in children. In: Fairbanks NF (ed): Snoring and Obstructive Sleep Apnea. New York, Raven Press, 1987. pp. 245-257.

Potsic WP, Wetmore RF: Sleep disorders and airway obstruction in children. *Otolaryngol Clin North Am* 23:651-663, 1990.

Siegel MB, Wetmore RF, Potsic WP, Handler SD, Tom LWC: Mandibular fractures in the pediatric patient. *Arch Otolaryngol Head Neck Surg* 117:533-536, 1991.

Stringer DA, Witzel MA: Comparison of multiview videofluoroscopy and nasopharyngoscopy in the assessment of velopharyngeal insufficiency. *Cleft Palate J* 26:88-92, 1989.

Stringer SP, Schaefer SD, Close LG: A randomized trial for outpatient management of peritonsillar abscess. *Arch Otolaryngol Head Neck Surg* 114:661-663, 1988.

Tom LWC, Anderson GJ, Womer RB, Wetmore RF, Handler SD, Potsic WP, Goldwein JW: Nasopharyngeal malignancies in children. *Laryngoscope* 102:509-514, 1992.

Wenig BM: Atlas of Head and Neck Pathology. Philadelphia, W.B. Saunders Co., 1993. pp. 105-199.

Wetmore RF. The oral cavity. In: Rudolph A (ed): Pediatrics, 19th ed. East Norwalk, Appleton and Lange, 1991. pp. 961-970.

CHAPTER 4

LARYNX AND TRACHEA

ANATOMY

The larynx is a funnel-shaped structures that serves as the connection between the pharynx and trachea (Fig. 4-1). It consists of a skeletal framework of articulated cartilages bound together by ligaments, membranes, and muscles. The thyroid cartilage is the anterior limit of the larynx, while the esophagus forms the posterior extent. The epiglottis is the most superior extension of the larynx and the cricoid cartilage (the only complete ring in the upper airway) marks its inferior boundary with the trachea. The subglottic space is defined as the area from the free edge of the true vocal cords to the inferior margin of the cricoid cartilage. It is the narrowest portion of the upper airway and is completely surrounded by the cricoid cartilage.

The paired arytenoid, corniculate, and cuneiform cartilages make up the remainder of the supporting skeleton of the larynx. In addition to extrinsic laryngeal muscles (the strap muscles and the inferior pharyngeal constrictor), five intrinsic muscles (cricothyroid, arytenoideus, thyroarytenoid) are responsible for the various functions of the larynx. The thyroarytenoid muscle, also called the vocalis muscle, forms the bulk of the true vocal cords that stretch from the inner surface of the midline of

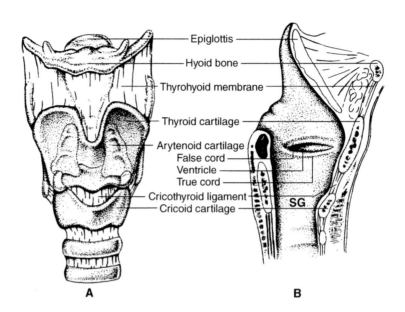

Figure 4–1. Larynx. (**A**) Frontal view of skeletal structure. (**B**) Sagittal view of internal structure. SG = subglottic space; AM = arytenoideus muscle. (From Potsic WP, Handler SD, Wetmore RF: Ear, Nose, Throat and Mouth. In: Rudolph A (ed). Pediatrics. 19th ed. Norwalk, CT, Appleton & Lange, 1991.)

the thyroid cartilage to the arytenoid cartilages posteriorly. The false vocal cords are folds of connective tissue located superior to and separated from the true vocal cords by the actions of the laryngeal ventricle. Movements of the vocal cords occur by the actions of the intrinsic muscles upon the arytenoid cartilages causing them to rotate and glide with respect to their cricoid articulations.

The intrinsic muscles of the larynx are innervated by the vagus nerve through the external division of the superior laryngeal nerve (supplying the cricothyroid muscle) and the recurrent laryngeal nerve (supplying the four remaining intrinsic muscles). All the intrinsic muscles adduct (i.e., close or approximate) the vocal cords except for the posterior cricoarytenoid muscle, which is the only one that abducts (opens) the cords. The action of the cricothyroid muscle is to tilt the thyroid cartilage on the cricoid cartilage and to tense the vocal cords.

Sensation to the larynx is supplied by the internal division of the superior laryngeal and sensory branches of the recurrent laryngeal nerves.

The blood supply to the larynx is through the superior thyroid branch of the external carotid artery. The larynx is lined throughout by a mucus-secreting ciliated epithelium except for the true vocal cords, which are covered by squamous epithelium.

The trachea extends from the inferior margin of the cricoid cartilage to its bifurcation into right and left bronchi at the carina. The right bronchus extends in a more-or-less straight line inferiorly from the trachea, while the left bronchi usually makes more of an obtuse angle with the trachea. This difference in angulation of the two bronchi accounts for the higher incidence of foreign bodies in the right side compared with the left. Approximately 20 C-shaped cartilage rings, open posteriorly, give structural support to the trachea. The trachea is lined with a mucus-setting ciliated epithelium and is innervated by the sensory branches of the recurrent laryngeal nerve.

PHYSIOLOGY

Respiration

One of the main functions of the larynx and trachea is respiration. The vocal cords must abduct to permit exchange or respiratory gases and must adduct to prevent aspiration. During inspiration, the larynx descends in the neck, by the action of the strap muscles, and the vocal cords abduct (Fig. 4-2). The larynx returns to its resting position during expiration. Any lesion that appears in the trachea or larynx such as a web, stenosis, or mass will interfere with the exchange of respiratory gases.

In the newborn infant, the larynx is approximately at the level of the second cervical vertebra. Thus, the epiglottis can be applied tightly to the posterior surface of the soft palate, effectively, sealing the oral cavity from the respiratory tract (Fig. 4-3). The newborn infant is an obligate nose-breather, capable of breathing and suckling simultaneously. During the first few months of life, the larynx begins its descent in the neck to its ultimate position opposite the fifth and sixth cervical vertebrae. When the epiglottis no longer makes this close contact with the soft palate, the infant ceases to be an obligate nose-breather.

The larynx is very important in the production of cough, a mechanism that is necessary for protecting and cleansing the lower airway. The sensation of a foreign body or of excess secretions is transmitted to the central nervous system by the sensory branches of the vagus nerve. A short

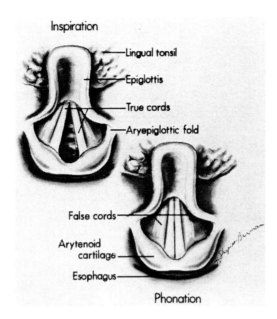

Inspiration

—Lingual tonsil

—Epiglottis

—True cords

—Aryepiglottic fold

False cords—

Arytenoid cartilage—

Esophagus—

Phonation

Figure 4–2. Endoscopic appearance of larynx in inspiration (vocal cords abducted) and phonation (vocal cords adducted). (From Potsic WP, Handler SD, Wetmore RF: Ear, Nose, Throat and Mouth. In: Rudolph A (ed). Pediatrics. 19th ed. Norwalk, CT, Appleton & Lange, 1991.)

inspiration is made and the vocal cords are then adducted. Intrathoracic pressure is raised by rapid elevation of the diaphragm; sudden abduction of the vocal cords results in a forceful expulsion of the foreign body or mucus. Dysfunction of the vagus nerve will impair this protective reflex and increase the incidence of aspiration.

Cleansing of the lower airway occurs through the larynx and trachea. Tracheal mucus and inhaled foreign particles are moved by the cilia and their mucus blanket superiorly through the larynx to the pharynx, where they are swallowed. Ciliary dysfunction or obstructive lesions in the larynx or trachea will decrease the efficiency of this function.

Another function of the larynx is to protect the airway from aspiration of food during deglutition. This sphincteric action of the larynx is phylogenetically its most primitive and, in many ways, its most important function. As swallowing is initiated, the larynx rises in the neck, the epiglottis folds posteriorly, and the true and false vocal cords come together in the midline. Although the epiglottis and false vocal cords help

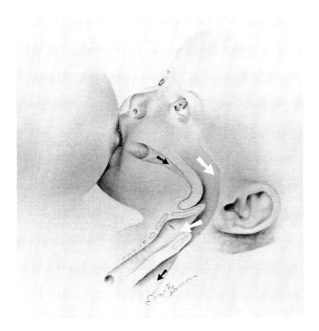

Figure 4–3. Diagram demonstrating intimate relationship between epiglottis and soft palate in an infant. White arrows illustrate the path of nasal airflow; black arrows show the route of fluids.

deflect the food bolus away from the laryngeal inlet, they are not really necessary for glottic competence. The true vocal cords themselves form the ultimate protective mechanism of the larynx.

Phonation

Normal phonation is dependent upon the approximation of normal vocal cords in the midline position (Fig. 4-2). Air is forced past the adducted vocal cords; thus, the cords vibrate synchronously, to form a tone. Vocal pitch is modified by alterations in the length, tension, and thickness of the vocal folds caused by the actions of the intrinsic laryngeal muscles. The pharynx and oral cavity then create the resonance chamber in which the tones are articulated into consonants and vowels. Conditions that prevent complete vocal cord approximation (e.g., unilateral vocal cord paralysis, vocal nodules, laryngeal masses) or that alter the mass of the vocal cords (e.g., edema, fibrosis) can result in a hoarse or breathy voice.

METHODS OF EXAMINATION

Direct and Indirect Examination

Examination of the larynx is often difficult in the younger child. Frequently, the tip of the epiglottis may be visualized when the tongue is protruded during the examination of the oropharynx. Indirect examination of the larynx can be performed using a laryngeal mirror or telescopic endoscope (*see* Chapter 3). Vocal cord mobility, the structure of the larynx, and the presence of laryngeal masses can usually be assessed in this manner in a cooperative child three years of age or older. In some instances, however, a general anesthetic is required to permit adequate inspection of the larynx. In these cases, direct laryngoscopy is performed so that laryngeal structure and function can be observed. Vocal cord mobility and airway dynamics are best evaluated using a flexible fiberoptic bronchoscope, while assessment and biopsy of laryngeal masses are performed through a standard laryngoscope. A portion of the upper tracheal rings can occasionally be seen on indirect laryngoscopy, but a general anesthetic is usually required to permit more complete direct examination of the upper trachea (tracheoscopy).

Radiologic Examination

Lateral and anterior-posterior plain radiographs of the neck can provide significant information about the larynx and upper trachea. While xeroradiographs, by virtue of their property of edge enhancement, offer more precise detail of the airway, the radiation exposure involved may make this a less desirable study. Computed tomography is very useful in examining the fine detail of laryngeal and tracheal structures. Fluoroscopic examination of the larynx is one method of evaluating the movement of the vocal cords during phonation and respiration. Vocal cord paralysis and laryngomalacia can often be identified in this manner. Contrast studies are also helpful in the evaluation of laryngeal function. A barium swallow can detect aspiration related to vocal cord paralysis, a posterior laryngeal cleft, or a tracheoesophageal fistula. A salivagram is a study in which the patient ingests a radioactive material followed by scanning of the lungs for evidence of aspiration. The new generation of rapid CT scans is able to provide the same detail seen with the laryngogram, yet with fewer difficulties.

COMMON COMPLAINTS

Hoarseness

Complete approximation of normal true vocal cords is necessary for the production of a normal voice. Any process that affects the structure or function of the vocal cords can lead to a harsh or hoarse voice. The most common cause of hoarseness in children is related to the laryngeal inflammation often associated with an *acute upper respiratory infection*. Edema of the vocal cords increases their mass thus, lowering the pitch of the voice and creating a hoarse sound. Poor approximation of the irregular free edges of the swollen vocal cords also contributes to the hoarse quality of the voice. The cause of the hoarseness is often evident with the presence of other symptoms of an upper respiratory infection, such as fever, rhinorrhea, cough, and sore throat. Indirect laryngoscopy is seldom necessary to confirm the diagnosis of laryngitis associated with upper respiratory infection. Treatment of upper respiratory infection consists of rest, fluids, antipyretics, and antimicrobials (if indicated). Voice rest will hasten the return of a normal voice following resolution of the upper respiratory infection. If the hoarseness persists despite adequate treatment, further evaluation is necessary.

Another common cause of hoarseness in children is *vocal cord nodules*. Vocal cord nodules (screamer's nodes) occur as a result of persistent vocal misuse or abuse by shouting, screaming, or even singing. These masses, are usually bilateral and occur at the junction of the anterior and middle one-thirds of the vocal cords (Fig. 4-4). The size of the nodules and the resultant hoarseness will often fluctuate, depending on the degree and amount of vocal abuse. If the diagnosis of vocal nodules is suspected, the child should be referred to an otolaryngologist for an indirect examination of the vocal cords. If this examination has confirmed the presence of vocal nodules, the child is referred to a voice or speech therapist. The therapist attempts to teach the child vocal techniques that will not strain the voice. Most vocal nodules will resolve after six to eight months of speech therapy. Occasionally, nodules that have become fibrotic as a result of long-standing vocal abuse may not respond to vocal therapy. The otolaryngologist may then perform a direct laryngoscopy and excise the vocal nodules. Generally, a normal voice will return after the nodules have been removed. The parents should be cautioned, however, that if the child returns to the poor speech habits that caused the problem, the nodules are likely to recur.

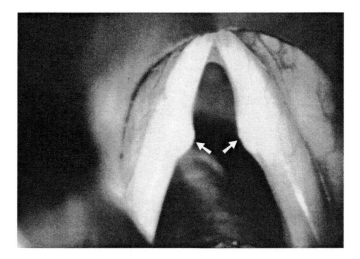

Figure 4–4. Endoscopic view of vocal cord nodules (arrows). (From Potsic WP, Handler SD, Wetmore RF: Ear, Nose, Throat and Mouth. In: Rudolph A (ed). Pediatrics. 19th ed. Norwalk, CT, Appleton & Lange, 1991.)

Small *vocal cord hemorrhages* can occur as a result of an episode of severe vocal abuse such as a singing session or cheering at a sports event. These can be seen on indirect laryngoscopy. With voice rest, the hoarseness that results will disappear as the hematomas resolve.

Chronic coughing and *throat-clearing* are uncommon causes of hoarseness. These actions involve forceful and repetitive adduction of the vocal cord, often resolving in thickened vocal cords and even nodule formation. After a complete evaluation of the child, therapy should be directed toward eliminating the condition that is requiring the throat-clearing (e.g., allergy, postnasal drip).

Less common causes of hoarseness include *vocal cord paralysis, trauma, laryngeal webs, polyps, cysts, foreign bodies,* and *neoplasms.* A complete examination of the upper airway is required in the evaluation of a child with hoarseness unrelated to an acute infection or vocal abuse. A history of trauma, intubation, or possible foreign body aspiration is helpful in directing the physician to the studies necessary to make the correct diagnosis. An otolaryngologist should be asked to perform a complete examination of the head and neck, including indirect laryngoscopy. Radiographs, including anterior-posterior and lateral views of the neck and chest, barium swallow, and fluoroscopy, are often useful in determining the cause of the hoarseness. Direct laryngoscopy, under a general anesthetic may be required to confirm the cause of the hoarseness and to perform the definitive treatment (e.g., biopsy a mass, remove a foreign body, excise a web).

Any process that affects the actual mass or bulk of the vocal cords can cause hoarseness as well. *Allergic edema* and *myxedema* of hypothyroidism are systemic causes of hoarseness. The diagnosis is made on the basis of the history and physical examination, including laryngoscopy. Treatment of the systemic condition usually results in the restoration of a normal voice.

Closely related to the symptom of hoarseness is that of a *breathy voice*. While incomplete and irregular approximation of the true vocal cords will produce a hoarse voice, a breathy voice will result if the vocal cords are separated during attempts at phonation. Vocal cord paralysis with inability to adduct the vocal cords completely is the most common cause of a breathy voice. Large granulomas or polyps in the larynx can also cause a breathy voice failing to allow the vocal cords to completely approximate.

Cough

Cough is a symptom that can accompany many conditions affecting the larynx. The cough may be an involuntary action caused by a reflex arc (involving sensory branches of the glossopharyngeal and vagus nerves and the motor branches of the recurrent laryngeal nerve), or it can be a voluntary action. Its function is to clear the trachea, larynx, or pharynx of mucus or any foreign material.

The most common cause of a cough is the laryngeal and pharyngeal inflammation associated with an upper respiratory infection. Other symptoms of *upper respiratory infection*, such as fever, sore throat, and rhinorrhea, will often accompany the cough. If the cough is a result of laryngeal edema in an upper respiratory infection, it will be dry and hacking. If excess mucus from the trachea or pharynx contacts the larynx, the cough produced to clear the airway is usually wet and productive. The cause of the cough in these cases is usually obvious with the presence of other signs of an upper respiratory infection. Physical examination will confirm the diagnosis by the demonstration of an erythematous pharynx and often tender cervical adenopathy. Radiographs of the sinuses and chest may be helpful in determining the possible sources of mucus that may contribute to the production of the cough. Treatment of the cough involves measures effective against the viral or bacterial upper respiratory infection with the addition of antitussive agents as required.

Patients who present with coughs that are paroxysmal, not obviously associated with an upper respiratory infection, or otherwise atypical deserve a more thorough evaluation. *Foreign body, neoplasms, allergy*, and *vocal nodules* are among the less common etiologies of a cough. Radiographs of the neck, sinuses, and chest should be obtained in the evaluation of these patients. An otolaryngologist should then be called upon to perform direct laryngoscopy and bronchoscopy in an effort to determine the cause of the cough and to begin proper treatment. Foreign body removal or biopsy of a suspicious lesion may be required.

Occasionally, a child will present with a history of paroxysms of coughing for which no cause can be determined. These coughing spells are usually disruptive to the child's functioning both in school and at home. If the history establishes that these spells do not occur when the child is eating or sleeping, a *psychogenic* cause for the cough must be strongly suggested. Usually a precipitating event can be elicited upon careful questioning of the child and his parents. A complete examination of the upper airway, including radiographs and indirect laryngoscopy, is necessary to rule out other causes of the cough before instituting counseling therapy.

A condition closely related to coughing is that of *constant throat-clearing*. This voluntary action is usually initiated by a child who has the feeling of a foreign body or excess mucus in or near the larynx. The act of throat-clearing is a short series of forceful expirations against tightly approximated vocal cords. This produces the vocalizations that accompany throat-clearing. Evaluation of the child with this symptoms is the same as that described for the atypical cough.

Stridor

The evaluation of the child with noisy respiration, or stridor, requires a careful history, a complete physical examination, and a knowledge of the functional anatomy of the upper airway. Normal respiratory efforts are usually not accompanied by audible sounds. If there is some point of obstruction in the airway requiring the normal respiratory volume of air to move faster to bypass the obstruction, turbulent airflow results, leading to noisy breathing. The stridor may originate from obstruction anywhere in the airway from the level of the anterior nares to the bronchi. Table 4-1 lists possible causes of stridor according to anatomic site.

The level of obstruction accounts for specific characteristics of the stridor that help localize the site of airway blockage. Obstruction of the nose (foreign body, polyp) or nasopharynx (enlarged adenoids, tumor) results in snoring or snorting sounds. This type of stridor is termed stertor. Because the passage of saliva and the flow of air are both impeded in pharyngeal obstruction, these patients often emit a gurgling type of noisy breathing. Laryngeal and subglottic obstruction is usually evidenced by high-pitched inspiratory stridor, while bronchial obstruction has characteristic expiratory wheezes. Tracheal obstruction usually presents with both inspiratory and expiratory stridor.

Esophageal foreign bodies can also present with stridor. The nature of the stridor depends on the location of the foreign body and degree of blockage that it is causing. Foreign bodies in the middle or distal portions of the esophagus can cause compression of the anteriorly placed trachea; these children will present with the high-pitched inspiratory and expiratory stridor characteristic of tracheal obstruction. If the foreign body is blocking the esophageal lumen and causing a backup of saliva up to the level of the pharynx, the child will demonstrate the gurgling stridor characteristic of pharyngeal obstruction.

The history is often very helpful in identifying the level of the obstruction and the source of the stridor. The child's parent should be questioned as to time of onset, duration, fluctuation, and any factors observed to alter the stridor. Stridor that does not appear until the child is four to six weeks old is most often laryngomalacia, while stridor evident at birth is more likely related to vocal cord paralysis, laryngeal cyst, or choanal atresia. Stridor that worsens with straining or crying may be caused by laryngomalacia or subglottic hemangioma. An antecedent history of an upper respiratory infection, neck trauma, or possible foreign body ingestion can point to the possible source of the stridor. A history of feeding problems in addition to the stridor suggests tracheoesophageal fistula, cleft larynx, vascular anomaly, or neurologic disorder as possible causes of the stridor. Episodes of drop attacks or of sudden collapse are usually indicative of a cardiovascular anomaly.

Much can be gained from a careful physical examination of the child who presents with stridor. The position that the child assumes can help the physician to identify the level of obstruction. Children with obstruction at the level of the larynx or above (e.g., epiglottis) usually hyperextend their neck in an attempt to straighten and maximize the upper airway. The phase of respiration in which the stridor occurs also helps localize the site of obstruction. Laryngeal obstruction is usually associated with inspiratory noise and a prolonged inspiratory phase of respiration, while bronchial obstruction has characteristic expiratory noises or wheezes and a similarly prolonged expiratory phase. Obstruction at the level of the trachea will often be associated with both inspiratory and expiratory stridor and respiratory phases that are approximately equal for inspiration and expiration.

Table 4-1 Causes of Stridor in Children According to Site of Obstruction

Nose and pharynx
Congenital anomalies
    Lingual thyroid
    Choanal atresia
    Craniofacial anomalies (Apert's, Down's, Pierre-Robin)
    Cysts (dermoid, thyroglossal)
    Macroglossia (Beckwith's syndrome)
    Encephalocele, glioma
Inflammatory
    Abscess (parapharyngeal, retropharyngeal, peritonsillar)
    Allergic polyps
    Adenotonsillar enlargement (acute infection, infectious
        mononucleosis)
Neoplasms (benign and malignant)
Adenotonsillar hypertrophy
Foreign body
Neurologic syndromes with poor tongue/pharyngeal muscle tone
Larynx
Congenital anomalies
    Laryngomalacia
    Web, cyst, laryngocele
    Cartilage dystrophy
    Cleft larynx
Inflammatory
    Croup
    Epiglottis
    Angioneurotic edema
    Miscellaneous (tuberculosis, fungus, diphtheria, sarcoidosis)
Vocal cord paralysis (multiple etiologies)
Trauma
    Intubation (laryngeal or subglottic edema, subglottic stenosis)
    Neck Trauma
    Foreign body
Neoplasm
    Subglottic hemangioma
    Laryngeal papilloma
    Cystic hygroma (neck)
    Malignant (e.g., rhabdomyosarcoma)
Laryngospasm (hypocalcemic tetany)

continued

Trachea and bronchi
    Congenital
        Vascular anomalies
        Webs, cysts
        Tracheal stenosis
        Tracheoesophageal fistula
    Foreign body (tracheal or esophageal)
    Neoplasm (benign and malignant)
        Tracheal
        Compression by neoplasm of adjacent structure (thyroid, thymus,
            esophagus)
    Trauma (tracheal stenosis secondary to intubation or tracheostomy)
    Inflammatory (bronchitis)
    Immunologic (asthma)

The presence and quality of the voice or cry can help identify laryngeal causes of stridor. A weak cry may be related to vocal cord disorders or to conditions involving poor pulmonary function (e.g., neuromuscular disorders). While laryngeal lesions are most often accompanied by voice changes, a normal voice does not rule out a laryngeal cause of stridor. For example, bilateral vocal cord paralysis most often presents with a normal voice in addition to its characteristic stridor.

Certain maneuvers can be performed during the physical examination and in effort to assess the functional anatomy of the upper airway and to determine the nature of the stridor. These actions may be both diagnostic and therapeutic with respect to the management of the child with stridor. If stridor is present immediately at birth, the first maneuver should be open the infant's mouth, pulling the mandible and tongue forward. If the stridor lessens, the obstruction is at the level of the larynx or higher. Nasal catheters should be passed to determine the patency of the nasopharyngeal airway and the possible presence of choanal atresia in any newborn infant in whom stridor is evident. In patients with choanal atresia, the placement of an oral airway will help confirm the diagnosis as well as relieve the obstruction. Pulling the mandible and tongue forward will often relieve the obstruction seen in Pierre-Robin sequence. Placing the child in the prone position can lessen the stridor in patients with laryngomalacia.

Radiographic studies are often invaluable in evaluating the child with stridor. Anterior-posterior and lateral views of the neck and chest are obtained to look for mass lesions and extrinsic compression of the airway. A barium swallow is useful in identifying vascular rings, tracheoesophageal fistulas, and neuromuscular disorders with aspiration and swallowing dysfunction. Fluoroscopy of the larynx can be obtained to evaluate vocal cord function. If a vascular ring is suspected, its presence may be confirmed by echocardiography or magnetic resonance angiography (MRA).

Indirect or direct laryngoscopy in the office setting is an important part of the examination of the child with stridor, especially of laryngeal origin. In a child older then three, indirect mirror examination of the larynx can assess vocal cord function or presence of a laryngeal mass. Similar information may be gained using a 90° rigid telescope or a flexible nasopharyngoscope.

The completeness and urgency of the evaluation of the child with stridor depends on the severity of obstruction and the presence of associated signs. If the infant with stridor is ventilating well and has no feeding problems, and no source for the obstruction can be found on physical or radiologic examination, the presumed diagnosis is laryngomalacia. The parents are reassured that the condition will most probably improve within the next few months. If the stridor is severe at the time of initial evaluation, or if it persists or worsens during a period of observation, further evaluation is indicated, and the child should be referred to an otolaryngologist. In addition to being able to perform a complete examination of the child's airway, the otolaryngologist is prepared to take the necessary steps to correct and/or bypass the cause of the stridor. Laryngoscopy and, often, bronchoscopy and esophagoscopy, may be required to determine the site of obstruction. Once the source of the stridor has been determined, efforts should be determined toward correcting the condition and relieving the respiratory distress. Rarely, this may include emergency intubation or tracheostomy.

The older child presenting with stridor requires the same careful history and complete physical examination as that described for an infant. As distinct from the infant in whom laryngomalacia is the most common cause of stridor, other problems such as adenotonsillar hypertrophy, foreign body, croup, and epiglottitis account for most cases of stridor in the older child. The otolaryngologist should assist in the evaluation and management of these cases.

CONGENITAL MALFORMATIONS

Laryngomalacia

Laryngomalacia is the most common cause of stridor in the infant. It is really not a malformation of the larynx, but a delay in maturation. The cartilage of infantile larynx is very flexible. As the child inspires, the laryngeal skeleton may not be stiff enough to keep the laryngeal lumen fully open. The epiglottis assumes a more pronounced infantile (omega) shape, and the aryepiglottic folds and false vocal cords are drawn into the laryngeal lumen. This results in a substantial narrowing of the lumen on aspiration that accounts for the high-pitched stridor heard in these infants. The stridor of laryngomalacia classically appears around the first month of life; before this time, the infant is unable to make a sufficiently strong inspiratory effort to create a stridorous sound. The child breathes more comfortably when in the prone position and when relaxed. When the child is agitated, and inspiration is more forceful, the stridor is usually worse. The diagnosis of laryngomalacia is often evident by the history and physical examination. Lateral neck and chest radiographs and a barium swallow are useful to rule out other causes for stridor. If the child, with a history consistent with laryngomalacia, has only infrequent episodes of stridor, is feeding well, and is gaining weight, and if radiologic investigation shows no abnormal findings, no further evaluation is necessary. The approach to this condition consists of close observation. As the child grows, the cartilage framework becomes more rigid in its support of the larynx, and the stridor disappears. Most children will outgrow this condition by their first birthday. If any of the following characteristics of stridor are present, further investigation is indicated: atypical stridor (present at birth or persisting after 8 to 12 months of age), worsening stridor, poor feeding and/or weight gain, and history of cyanotic or apneic episodes. In these instances, an otolaryngologist should be called upon to perform direct laryngoscopy to confirm the diagnosis of laryngomalacia and to rule out other causes of stridor. While most patients can be managed expectantly, in some case of laryngomalacia severe respiratory distress or feeding difficulties may necessitate airway intervention with intubation of tracheotomy.

Vocal Cord Paralysis

Vocal cord paralysis is the second most common congenital disorder of the larynx and one of the most common causes of stridor in the newborn. Causes and treatment of this problem are discussed in a later section. (*See* page 138.)

Subglottic Stenosis

Congenital subglottic stenosis is another cause of stridor in the neonate. Narrowing of the subglottic airway can occur secondary to any one or combination of the following characteristics: abnormally high position of the first tracheal ring with respect to the cricoid cartilage, decreased size of the cricoid ring, or excess soft tissue contained within the cricoid ring. If the presence of the subglottic stenosis is suspected on clinical or radiographic grounds, the otolaryngologist should be consulted to confirm the diagnosis by endoscopic evaluation. There is considerable controversy regarding the treatment of this condition. Children with only mild stenosis, resulting in minimal or no symptoms, require no active treatment. Only stenosis sufficient to produce signs of significant respiratory distress, bradycardia, poor weight gain, cyanotic episodes, or recurrent pulmonary infections requires treatment. The most conservative management involves performing a tracheostomy and allowing the subglottic space to widen as the child grows. Moderate to severe stenosis may be treated surgically with either a cricoid split or laryngotracheoplasty.

Laryngeal Webs, Cysts, and Laryngocele

Glottic webs can occur as a result of incomplete breakdown of the epithelial diaphragm that covers the laryngeal inlet during embryonic life. Abnormal voice and, in more severe cases, stridor, and respiratory distress can be the presenting signs. Intubation or tracheostomy can be life saving in the more complete glottic webs. *Tracheal webs* are uncommon; the symptoms depend upon the degree of obstruction they produce. *Congenital cysts* of the larynx usually occur in the supraglottic region and occasionally in the subglottic space. They arise from the mucus-secreting epithelium of the larynx. Presenting symptoms include stridor and sometimes hoarseness. Simple aspiration or marsupialization of the cyst is the recommended treatment. *Laryngoceles* are epithelial-lined diverticula that originate in the laryngeal ventricle. They can present internally in the laryngeal lumen with airway obstruction or externally as a neck mass. Total excision of the cyst is the treatment of choice. If the presence of any of these congenital anomalies is suspected, an otolaryngologist should be consulted for examination of the upper airway and treatment of the specific condition.

Laryngotracheoesophageal Defects

Incomplete formation of the laryngotracheal septum can leave abnormal connections between the food and air passages. *Posterior laryngeal clefts* range from a slight deepening of the interarytenoid notch to a complete posterior cleft of the larynx and upper trachea. The child will present with a history of aspiration, recurrent pulmonary infections, failure to thrive, hoarseness, and occasionally upper airway obstruction. The cleft is often difficult to demonstrate radiographically or endoscopically. Surgical repair of the cleft is the treatment of choice and should be performed soon after the diagnosis is confirmed. Tracheostomy may be required in the treatment of some cases.

Tracheoesophageal fistula, with or without esophageal atresia, is an uncommon condition, occurring in approximately 1 in 4,500 live births. The diagnosis of tracheoesophageal fistula will usually depend on the presence of associated esophageal anomalies. The child with the most common type of tracheoesophageal fistula, consisting of esophageal atresia and a distal tracheoesophageal fistula, will present with immediate regurgitation and aspiration of feedings, often accompanied by cyanosis. The abdomen is usually distended with air, and respiratory distress progresses with continued aspiration of saliva and feedings. The diagnosis is confirmed by contrast radiographs. Surgical repair by a general or thoracic surgeon should be undertaken as soon as possible, preferably within the first few days of life. The H type of tracheoesophageal fistula may not be discovered until the child is several months of age. The child will usually present with a history of recurrent episodes of aspiration pneumonia, coughing, and choking while feeding. Surgical closure of the fistula should be performed as soon as the diagnosis is confirmed by radiographic or endoscopic techniques. Tracheostomy and gastrostomy may be required in the management of difficult cases of tracheoesophageal fistula associated with significant respiratory distress or a long segment of esophageal atresia.

Vascular Anomalies

Several vascular anomalies in the neck and thorax can cause respiratory obstruction by compression of the trachea. These include, in descending order of occurrence, *right aortic arch, double aortic arch, anomalous (retroesophageal) right subclavian artery,* and *anomalous innominate artery.* The diagnosis of these conditions is often suggested by the history of feeding problems and some degree of respiratory distress in a newborn. A vascular anomaly with only minimal compression of the trachea may cause significant symptoms concomitant with an upper respiratory infection. Radiographs are extremely useful in confirming the diagnosis of a vascular lesion. Diagnostic studies include plain view of the chest and neck, barium swallow, echocardiography and MRA. The management of these anomalies is undertaken by a cardiovascular surgeon.

INFECTIOUS DISEASES

Viral Infections

Viral laryngitis is often a component of the common upper respiratory infection described in Chapters 2 and 3. The same viruses have been implicated as the causative organisms of the laryngitis. Laryngeal involvement is indicated by a hoarse, raspy voice. This is related to edema of the vocal cords, secondary to the viral inflammation. Airway obstruction is rare in viral laryngitis. Symptomatic treatment with humidification, antipyretics, analgesics, throat gargles, and voice rest is recommended while the disease runs its natural course.

When the viral infection involves the subglottic space, a more serious clinical problem appears. *Laryngotracheobronchitis* (*croup*) is a common, and potentially life-threatening, infection that occurs in early childhood. Children between the ages of one and five years are involved most frequently, and there appears to be a seasonal predominance in the fall and winter months. While, as the name implies, the viral infection affects a large portion of the respiratory tract, it is the involvement of the subglottic space that causes the morbidity and mortality associated with croup. Subglottic edema is responsible for the characteristic inspiratory stridor and the brassy or barky cough. *Parainfluenza* viruses account for most croup infections.

The diagnosis of croup is most often made on the basis of the history and physical examination. The child usually presents with a history of upper respiratory infection, low-grade fever, progressive difficulty breathing, stridor, and a characteristic brassy or barky cough. Anterior-posterior and lateral neck radiographs will demonstrate subglottic narrowing (Fig. 4-5).

While most children are adequately managed at home with humidification and antipyretics, some patients may require more intensive therapy. Children who become fatigued from the work of breathing (i.e., have significant suprasternal, intercostal, and subcostal retractions), or who demonstrate cyanosis or hypoxia require hospitalization and management by a team including pediatricians, otolaryngologists, and critical care specialists. Supportive care with humidification and hydration should be started immediately. Many centers routinely employ racemic epinephrine delivered by nebulizer to reduce the subglottic edema in order to reduce the airway obstruction. Antimicrobial therapy probably does not play a role in the treatment of this viral illness. The use of corticosteroids in the management of croup is controversial. While some studies have shown significant improvement in the symptoms of patients treated with corti-

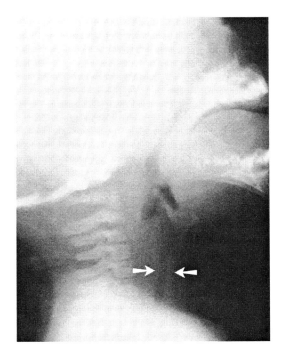

A

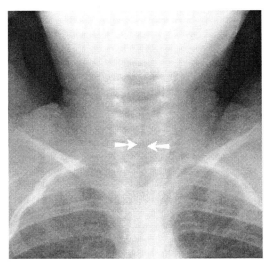

B

Figure 4–5. Croup (laryngotracheobronchitis). (**A**) Lateral neck radiograph demonstrating narrowing of subglottic airway (arrow). (**B**) Posterior-anterior chest radiograph showing symmetric narrowing (pencil or steeple sign) of the subglottic airway (arrows).

costeroids, other investigators have found such treatment to have no effect.

If the patient becomes excessively fatigued or the obstruction worsens causing hypoxia, hypercarbia, bradycardia, or tachypnea, an artificial airway is required. Nasotracheal intubation is usually employed first. Since the lumen of the airway is narrowed secondary to the acute infection, the endotracheal tube should be 0.5 mm to 1.0 mm smaller than what would be an appropriate tube for the same child under normal circumstances. The endotracheal tube must be managed carefully to avoid the complication of subglottic stenosis. An air leak should be detectable around the endotracheal tube on positive-pressure ventilation, by bag or ventilator, indicating that the tube is not applying a significant pressure on the surrounding tracheal and subglottic mucosa. Tracheostomy should be performed if the nasotracheal tube cannot be placed, or if it fits too tightly within the subglottic space. The artificial airway is usually left in place for three to five days and removed when the subglottic edema has decreased enough to allow normal respiration. This can be determined by an increasing air leak around the tube or by endoscopic examination of the subglottic space.

Because multiple agents can cause croup, a single episode does not grant immunity from further recurrences. Recurrent episodes of croup, especially in a child under six months of age, however, should alert the clinician to the possibility of some predisposing cause, such as congenital subglottic stenosis or the presence of a foreign body. The child should be referred to an otolaryngologist for endoscopic examination of the airway.

Bacterial Infections

Bacterial *laryngitis* does occur but it is not nearly as common as its viral counterpart. It is also very difficult to distinguish bacterial laryngitis on clinical grounds from a similar infection of viral etiology. Etiologic agents responsible for bacterial laryngitis include *Staphylococcus* and *Hemophilus influenzae*. Treatment consists of the same measures recommended for viral laryngitis, with the addition of the appropriate antimicrobial agents.

Diphtheria is of historical interest in the United States today. The diphtheria membrane covers the larynx and can compromise the laryngeal airway and thereby cause acute airway obstruction requiring either endoscopic removal of the membrane or tracheostomy, or both, in addition to antimicrobial therapy.

Tuberculosis of the larynx can occur as an isolated infection, but it is most often found in association with a generalized pulmonary infection.

The larynx is red and granular, causing hoarseness and a sore throat. Diagnosis is made on the basis of laryngeal culture or biopsy.

Bacterial infection of the supraglottic larynx can cause a symptom complex with potentially life-threatening airway obstruction. *Epiglottitis* — more appropriately termed *supraglottitis* — is an infection of the supraglottic larynx caused most often by *H. influenzae* type B. Less commonly, *Streptococcus, Staphylococcus,* and other bacteria have been implicated in this disease that primarily affects children between two and five years of age. The history is usually one of recent onset of fever, drooling, sore throat, and airway distress. Dyspnea may progress rapidly to complete airway obstruction and asphyxiation. The mechanism of this acute airway obstruction in the epiglottis is unclear; laryngospasm and acute blockage of the narrowed airway with inspissated mucus have both been suggested as possible causes.

The diagnosis of epiglottitis is often suggested by the history and may be confirmed on the basis of physical examination. Affected children are toxic, anxious, and usually sitting upright with their chins extended in an effort to maximize the airway. The cherry-red, swollen epiglottis can sometimes be discovered during examination of the child when the tongue blade is placed on the posterior aspect of the tongue. Extreme care must be taken during this part of the examination not to induce acute airway obstruction. Attempts should be made to keep the child as calm as possible and to minimize stimulation of the pharynx, since both agitation and instrumentation of the pharynx are reported to increase the potential for acute airway obstruction. Appropriate equipment and personnel trained to perform either intubation or tracheostomy, or both, should be present when examining a child with possible epiglottitis. Lateral neck radiographs are helpful in confirming the clinical suspicion of epiglottitis and in differentiating this from croup. A large, swollen epiglottis and supraglottic structures confirm the diagnosis (Fig. 4-6).

Proper management of the child with epiglottitis requires close cooperation of the pediatrician, otolaryngologist, and anesthesiologist. Once the diagnosis is made, an artificial airway is usually placed to prevent catastrophic airway obstruction. Considerable controversy exists in the literature concerning the relative safety and efficacy of nasotracheal intubation versus tracheostomy for airway management in epiglottitis. The choice of airway management is probably one that is best decided by local factors such as staff training and available facilities. Treatment with ampicillin and chloramphenicol or a third generation cephalosporin is begun immediately, later modified by blood or laryngeal culture results. The artificial airway is removed once evidence of decreased supraglottic swelling is present. A repeat laryngoscopy or lateral

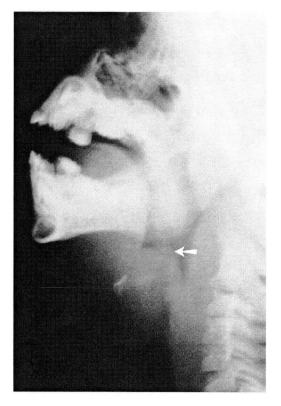

Figure 4–6. Lateral neck radiograph demonstrating swollen epiglottis (arrows) in a patient with acute supraglottitis.

neck radiograph can be used to determine whether the laryngeal lumen has improved enough to permit adequate ventilation. Epiglottitis (in contradistinction to croup) rarely, if ever, recurs. The incidence of epiglottitis has been shown to have decreased since the introduction of the conjugated *H. influenza* vaccine.

Fungal Infections

Fungal infections of the larynx are uncommon and are usually a part of a more generalized disease process. *Histoplasma capsulatum* and *Coccidioides immitis* are two organisms that have been identified in laryngeal biopsies or cultures from patients who demonstrated a nonspecific laryngitis. Parenteral treatment with antifungal agents is the treatment of choice. Tracheostomy may be required to protect the airway in some affected patients.

NEOPLASMS

Benign Neoplasms

The most common neoplasm of the larynx in children is the *laryngeal papilloma*. Though to be a viral-induced neoplasm, it has a predilection for the upper aerodigestive tract and the larynx in particular. A large body of literature suggests an association between laryngeal papillomas in the child and veneral condylomata in the mother. The disease usually makes its presentation in the child between two and five years of age with persistent or worsening hoarseness and, occasionally, airway obstruction. A lateral neck radiograph may demonstrate the presence of papillomas in the larynx. If the papillomas are suspected as the source of hoarseness in a child, an otolaryngologist should be consulted to perform the indirect or direct laryngoscopy required to confirm the diagnosis. The course of the disease is characterized by multiple cycles of growth and regression, until a spontaneous remission occurs, usually around puberty. None of the recommended treatments, which include surgical excision, laser excision, cryotherapy, ultrasound, systemic antiviral agents such as interferon or acyclovir, or topical agents such as podophyllin or antimetabolites, has been shown to cure this disease. The goal in managing these patients is to maintain a good voice and an unobstructed airway by repeated excision of the papillomas. In some patients, however, despite all efforts to keep the larynx clear, rapid growth of papillomas causes airway obstruction sufficient to require a tracheostomy.

Hemangiomas may occur in the larynx, primarily in the subglottic area. These are often associated with other cutaneous hemangiomas but can occur as isolated lesions. As with most juvenile hemangiomas, these lesions present in the third to sixth month of life and can enlarge over several months to cause significant airway obstruction. Episodes of stridor may be precipitated by an upper respiratory infection. Hemangiomas appear as posterior subglottic masses on lateral neck radiographs, but the diagnosis usually must be confirmed by laryngoscopy. Since many hemangiomas in infancy tend to involute after a period of growth (i.e., during the first one to two years of life), close observation has been advocated as the treatment of those lesion which are causing minimal symptoms (i.e., only mild stridor with upper respiratory infection, no feeding problems, good weight gain). If the child is in severe, persistent, or recurrent respiratory distress, intervention is indicated; an otolaryngologist should be consulted to assist the primary physician in the management of these difficult cases. The most conservative mode of therapy involves tracheostomy to protect the airway while awaiting the expected involution of the lesion. Corticosteroids have been used to induce early involution of the hemangiomas, but protracted use of these drugs can have serious side effects, such as growth retardation, in these young patients. Surgical excision of subglottic hemangiomas had been both difficult and dangerous until the introduction of the CO_2 laser, which permits safe removal with minimal risk of airway obstruction or hemorrhage. Radiation therapy has also been successful in shrinking hemangiomas; nevertheless, the risk of irradiation-induced malignancy makes this an undesirable treatment modality for a benign neoplasm.

Malignant Neoplasms

Malignant neoplasms of the larynx are rare. They include *rhabdomyosarcoma, chondrosarcoma*, and *lymphoma*. These lesions present with varying degrees of hoarseness and respiratory obstruction. If a laryngeal malignancy is suspected, an otolaryngologist should be asked to perform indirect and direct laryngoscopy to confirm the laryngeal problem and to obtain tissue for histologic identification of the tumor. Treatment and prognosis are dependent upon the nature and extent of the neoplasm.

ALLERGIC CONDITIONS

The larynx is sensitive to the same allergens that affect other parts of the upper aerodigestive tract. When the mucosa of the larynx is involved, edema of the vocal cords results in a hoarse voice and a dry, scratchy feeling in the throat. The larynx may also be irritated by an allergic postnasal drip. Treatment of allergic manifestations in the larynx includes avoidance of the offending allergen, as well as systemic antihistamines, humidification, systemic or aerosol corticosteroids, and desensitization.

Spasmodic croup is thought to be allergic in origin. In cases of spasmodic croup, the child will often be well when going to bed, but will wake up in the middle of the night with a barky cough and mild inspiratory stridor. The condition responds to humidification. Occasionally, a short (one to two dose) course of corticosteroids may be helpful. The child is then usually able to go back to sleep without stridor. The next day the child is well again, but the same episode is repeated on two or three successive nights. The repetitive nature of this problem, along with the absence of any signs of an upper respiratory infection, separate this entity from acute infectious croup.

TRAUMA

Laryngeal trauma can occur in a variety of ways. Blunt or penetrating injuries of the larynx can result in mucosal lacerations, laryngeal hematomas, vocal cord paralysis, or fractures of the thyroid and cricoid cartilages. *Endotracheal intubation* can also cause mucosal lacerations, vocal cord paralysis, or dislocation of the arytenoid cartilage. Laryngeal edema, mucosal ulceration, webs, granulomas, and stenosis are sequelae of long-term intubation. Proper treatment requires prompt recognition of the presence and nature of a laryngeal injury, as well as protection of the airway. Patients with laryngeal trauma present with varying degrees of neck pain, hoarseness, hemoptysis, and airway obstruction. Physical examination of a child with blunt trauma can demonstrate anterior neck tenderness, crepitance, and absence of the normal prominence of the thyroid cartilage (Adam's apple). An otolaryngologist should be consulted to perform indirect or direct examination of the larynx. It may be necessary to intervene with intubation, tracheostomy, and surgical exploration of these laryngeal injuries. Late sequelae of laryngeal injury such as stenosis, webs, and granulomas are marked by varying degrees of hoarseness and stridor. These patients require endoscopic evaluation and treatment directed to the specific problem.

Subglottic stenosis is a serious complication that can occur as a result of endotracheal intubation in children. Mucosal edema followed by ulceration occurs as the subglottic mucosa is compressed by the pressure of a tight-fitting endotracheal tube against the encircling cricoid cartilage; the resultant chondritis and/or mucosal fibrosis can then narrow the subglottic lumen. Such factors as placement of too large an endotracheal tube, inadequate fixation of the tube, prolonged length of intubation, the use of a cuffed endotracheal tube have all been found to increase the risk of developing subglottic stenosis. Subglottic stenosis should be suspected in any child who is unable to be extubated after a period of endotracheal intubation. The otolaryngologist should be consulted to perform the endoscopy required to confirm the diagnosis. Subglottic stenosis is best avoided by minimizing predisposing factors and by preventing its occurrence. Once the complication of stenosis has occurred, treatment is the same as that described for subglottic stenosis of congenital origin.

Ingestion of *caustic substances* can cause severe burns of the larynx and pharynx resulting in airway obstruction secondary to the burn edema. Laryngeal burns should be suspected in the child in whom hoarseness or stridor develops after caustic ingestion. The child should be hospitalized and the airway monitored. If signs of respiratory distress (tachypnea, severe stridor) occur, the child should be taken to the operating room for endoscopic evaluation before an artificial airway, usually a tracheotomy, is placed.

Vocal nodules (screamer's nodules) occur as a result of persistent vocal misuse or abuse by shouting, screaming, or even singing. This problem is discussed in detail in the section on common complaints. (*See* page 117.)

Gastroesophageal reflux can occur up to the level of the larynx and cause inflammation of the arytenoids and the supraglottic structures. Some investigators believe that this reflux may lead to laryngospasm and might therefore be a possible cause of sudden infant death syndrome (SIDS). Monitoring of the pH is usually required to confirm the diagnosis of reflux. Indirect or direct laryngoscopy will reveal the erythematous arytenoids characteristic of laryngeal inflammation secondary to reflux.

Foreign Bodies

Foreign bodies may become trapped in the laryngeal inlet, causing acute upper airway obstruction. The child will usually present with severe coughing, hoarseness, and significant respiratory distress. If the child is able to phonate, air is moving through his larynx and he is only partially obstructed. "Back slaps" or the Heimlich maneuver should not be performed in these children, since this may cause the foreign body to lodge more firmly in the larynx and convert a partial obstruction into a complete one. The child should be transported immediately to the hospital, where an otolaryngologist can perform a direct laryngoscopy to remove the foreign body. If the child is unable to speak, the airway may be totally obstructed by the foreign body. For this true emergency condition, back slaps or the Heimlich maneuver may be life saving.

Foreign bodies that pass the larynx and lodge in the trachea or proximal bronchi can present problems both in diagnosis and in management. Usually a history of coughing or choking on food (most often a peanut, raw carrot, etc.) or a toy is obtained. The child is usually in no acute distress but demonstrates a mild cough or wheeze. Inspiratory and expiratory stridor are characteristic of tracheal foreign bodies. Unilateral wheezes and decreased, or even absent, breath sounds are often seen with unilateral bronchial obstruction. Since most of the foreign bodies are radiolucent, they are not identifiable on radiographs. However, a difference in aeration of the lungs will often help detect the presence and identify the site of a bronchial obstruction. Volume decrease, atelectasis, and infiltrate are often seen on plain chest films. Hyperaeration (air trapping) secondary to a ball-valve effect of the foreign body are best seen by comparing inspiration and expiration films (Fig. 4-7). If the child does not cooperate to obtain these views, right and left lateral decubitus films can often demonstrate the same phenomena. A normal chest radiograph, however, does not rule out the possibility of a foreign body. If a foreign body is sus-

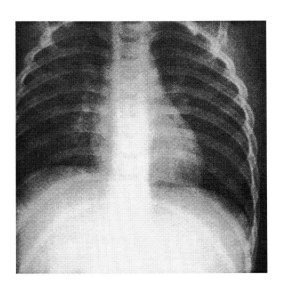

A

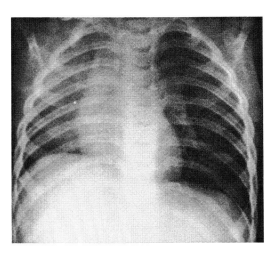

B

Figure 4–7. Foreign body of the left bronchus. **(A)** Inspiratory film is normal. **(B)** Expiratory film demonstrates hyperaeration and air trapping (left).

pected on the basis of the history or clinical or radiographic examination, otolaryngologic consultation should be obtained to perform the endoscopy necessary for its prompt and safe removal.

METABOLIC DISORDERS

A variety of metabolic disorders may become manifest by laryngeal abnormalities. *Myxedema fluid* (related to the hypothyroidism), *amyloid*, or *mucopolysaccharide* can accumulate in the vocal cords, causing a hoarse voice and, rarely, airway obstruction. Tetany associated with *hypocalcemia* can result in laryngospasm and acute upper airway obstruction. Vocal cord paresis or paralysis may occur secondary to the neuropathy of *diabetes mellitus* or as a result of *heavy metal poisoning*. In each of these cases, hoarseness or stridor are the presenting symptoms and require otolaryngologic assistance for the endoscopic examination necessary to confirm the diagnosis.

INFLAMMATORY DISORDERS

Inflammatory disorders uncommonly affect the larynx. *Cricoarytenoid arthritis* can occur in children with juvenile rheumatoid arthritis. Hoarseness and sore throat are the presenting symptoms. The diagnosis is confirmed by endoscopic demonstration of an inflamed and immobile arytenoid. Treatment is usually medical, although arytenoidectomy is occasionally required in cases of bilateral involvement with airway obstruction. *Sarcoidosis* has been described in the larynx, causing hoarseness and a nonspecific laryngitis. Usually this is associated with generalized sarcoidosis of the upper airway. The diagnosis is made by the demonstration of noncaseating granulomas on a biopsy of a lesion in the larynx, trachea, or a mediastinal lymph node. There is no treatment for the idiopathic disease, although corticosteroids are useful for symptomatic relief. Tracheostomy may be required in cases of severe airway obstruction.

VOCAL CORD PARALYSIS

The proper management of patients with vocal cord paralysis requires a complete history and physical examination and close cooperation between the primary practitioner and the consulting otolaryngologist. The possible causes of vocal cord paralysis in children are listed in Table 4-2. Unilateral recurrent laryngeal nerve paralysis results in assumption of a midline or slightly abducted position in the affected cord. On inspiration, the normal vocal cord abducts completely, creating an airway adequate for all except the most strenuous exercise. Symptoms of unilateral vocal cord paralysis are often so mild that the disorder goes unnoticed. Stridor is characteristically absent in these patients. The cry may be weak or hoarse if the vocal cords do not approximate completely. A breathy voice results when there is a large gap between the cords during phonation. The voice usually returns to normal as the unaffected vocal cord compensates for the paralyzed cord. Aspiration may occur if the normal cord fails to accomplish the compensation for the paralyzed cord and if there is incomplete laryngeal closure during deglutition. Superior laryngeal nerve injury results in paralysis of the cricothyroid muscle on that side. Decreased tension of that vocal cord accounts for the slight decrease

Table 4-2   Etiologies of Vocal Cord Paralysis

Congenital
    Central nervous system or disease
    Birth trauma to head or neck
    Cysts (neck or chest)
Neoplasm (intracranial, cervical, thoracic)
    Benign
    Malignant
Inflammatory
    Infection (viral)
    Degenerative disease (rheumatoid arthritis)
Metabolic disease
    Diabetes mellitus
    Heavy-metal poisoning (arsenic, lead)
Trauma (including surgery)
    Blunt or penetrating (neck, head, chest)
    Intubation
Neurological
    Central nervous system disease
    Neuromuscular disease (e.g., myasthenia gravis)
Vascular
    Cardiovascular anomalies
    Cardiac failure (left heart enlargement)

in vocal range characteristics of superior laryngeal paralysis. Treatment is seldom required for unilateral vocal cord paralysis because of the potential for return of function or compensation by the other cord. Teflon is occasionally injected into the paralyzed vocal cord to improve the voice or to prevent aspiration if symptoms persist 6 to12 months after the initial injury.

Bilateral recurrent laryngeal paralysis is usually characterized by marked airway obstruction and a good voice; both vocal cords are paralyzed in the midline or slightly abducted position. Management of bilateral vocal cord paralysis requires prompt intervention, usually tracheostomy, to relieve the airway obstruction. If the cause of the vocal paralysis is treatable (e.g., posterior craniectomy for Arnold-Chiari malformation) or resolves (e.g., Guillain-Barre syndrome), the vocal cords may regain mobility and permit decannulation. If the paralysis is permanent, an adequate airway may be created by any of several procedures that lateralize one of the cords in order to permit decannulation. An improvement in airway, however, may be at the cost of voice quality.

EMERGENCY AIRWAY INTERVENTION (TRACHEOSTOMY)

In the vast majority of cases of airway obstruction, there is ample time for an orderly approach to management. This includes medical therapy, intubation, and transfer to the operating room for emergency endoscopy, intubation, or tracheostomy. In rare cases the child is totally obstructed, and techniques such as the Heimlich maneuver and emergency laryngoscopy in the emergency room fail to alleviate the obstruction. In these cases, a true emergency tracheostomy in the emergency room becomes necessary. This is a very rare occurrence and should only be attempted when all other attempts have failed to relieve the upper airway obstruction and the child is moribund.

The child should be placed on this back and a rolled-up sheet placed under his shoulders to help extend his neck. The physician should identify the trachea and stabilize it with two fingers of his left hand. The thyroid cartilage and the suprasternal notch should be identified. Local anesthesia is waste of precious time and unnecessary if the child is unconscious. A vertical incision is made in the skin of the neck from the thyroid cartilage to the suprasternal notch. Since the midline contains few blood vessels, the incision is usually bloodless. The trachea is identified by its transverse cartilaginous rings and is entered in a vertical manner. Care must be taken to stay in the midline and not to incise the posterior tracheal wall. The tracheostomy (or endotracheal) tube is inserted into the trachea and fixed in place with ties or tape. Once the tube is secured and the patient stabilized, he should be taken to the operating room, where the otolaryngologist can examine the upper airway to determine the cause of airway obstruction. The tracheostomy site should be inspected and bleeding vessels ligated. If the tracheostomy tube is close to (or through) the cricoid cartilage, the stoma should be relocated to the cervical trachea in order to avoid the complication of subglottic stenosis.

SUGGESTED READINGS

Banks, Potsic WP: Elusive unsuspected foreign bodies in the tracheobronchial tree. *Clin Pediatr* 16:31-35, 1977.

Cotton RT: Pediatric laryngeal stenosis. *J Pediatr Surg* 19:699-704, 1984.

Denneny JC, Handler SD: Membranous laryngotracheobronchitis (LTB). *Pediatrics* 70:705-707, 1982.

Fearon B, MacRae D: Laryngeal papillomatosis in children. *J Otolaryngol* 5:493-496, 1976.

Garfinkle TS, Handler SD: Hemangiomas of the head and neck in children: Guide to management. *J Otolaryngol* 9:439-450, 1980.

Handler SD: Diagnosis and management of maxillo-facial injuries . In: Athletic Injuries to the Head, Neck and Face. Torg J (ed). Philadelphia, Lea and Febiger. 1982, pp. 223-244.

Handler SD, Raney RB: Management of neoplasms of the head and neck in children. I. Benign tumors. *Head Neck Surg* 3:395-405, 1981.

Holinger PH, Brown WT: Congenital webs, cysts, laryngoceles, and other anomalies of the larynx. *Ann Otol Rhinol Laryngol* 76:744-752, 1967.

Kessler A, Wetmore RF, Marsh RR: Childhood epiglottitis in recent years. *Int J Pediatr Otorhinolaryngol* 25:155-162, 1993.

Lepizia B, Osler FA, Cummings CW, et al: A prospective randomized study to determine the efficacy of steroids in the management of croup. *J Pediatr* 94:194- 196, 1979.

McGovern RH, Fitz-Hugh GS, Edgeman LJ: The hazards of endotracheal intubation. *Ann Otol Rhinol Laryngol* 80:556-564, 1971.

Montgomery WW: Surgery of the Upper Respiratory System, Vol. 2. Philadelphia, Lea and Febiger. 1973, pp. 315-372.

Papsidero MJ, Pashley NRT: Acquired stenosis of the upper airway in neonates. *Ann Otol Rhinol Laryngol* 89:512-514, 1980.

Raney RB, Handler SD: Management of neoplasms of the head and neck in children. II Malignant tumors. *Head Neck Surg* 3:500-507, 1981.

Rosin DF, Handler SD, Potsic WP, Wetmore RF, Tom LWC: Vocal cord paralysis in children. *Laryngoscope* 100:1174-1179, 1990.

Strong RM, Passy V: Endotracheal intubation — Complications in neonates. *Arch Otolaryngol* 103:329-335, 1977.

Wetmore RF, Handler SD: Epiglottitis: Evolution in management during the last decade. *Ann Otol Rhinol Laryngol* 88:822-826, 1979.

Wetmore RF, Handler SD, Potsic WP: Pediatric tracheostomy: Experience during the past decade. *Ann Otol Rhinol Laryngol* 91:628-632, 1982.

CHAPTER 5

NECK AND ASSOCIATED STRUCTURES

ANATOMY

Contained within the neck are parts of several vital organ systems which are responsible for many of the disease processes that present in the head and neck. The complex anatomy of the various structures within the neck may be appreciated by a cross-sectional view (Fig. 5-1).

The neck is divided into several components by condensations of connective tissue. The presence of these space helps explain the spread of infectious and neoplastic processes both within and through the neck. Between the visceral compartment, which contains the esophagus, trachea, and thyroid gland, and the prevertebral layer of fascia lies the retropharyngeal space. This potential space extends from the base of the skull as far as the mediastinum, creating a natural path for infections of the head and neck to spread into the chest and cause such inflammations as mediastinitis. The parapharyngeal space is located lateral to the pharynx and medial to the mandible. Infectious organisms entering this space from the visceral compartment have access to the vascular sheath as a means of further spread.

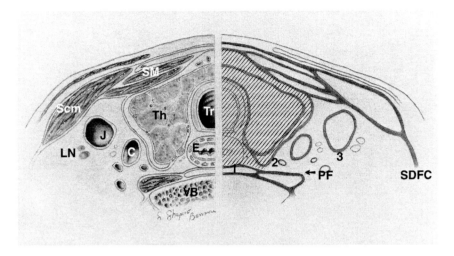

Figure 5–1. Cross-sectional view of the neck at the level of the upper trachea.

SDCF = Superficial layer of Deep Cervical Fascia

SM = Strap muscle	**Scm** = Sternocleidomastoid muscle
J = Jugular vein	**C** = Carotid artery
Th = Thyroid gland	**Tr** = Trachea
E = Esophagus	**LN** = Lymph nodes
VB = Vertebral body	**PF** = Prevertebral fascia
1 = Retropharyngeal space	**2** = Parapharyngeal space
3 = Carotid (Vascular sheath	**Shaded area** = Visceral compartment

The superficial and pretracheal layers of the deep cervical fascia are separated by a complex network of lymphatic channels that drain the structures of the head and neck. The neural structures traversing the neck include the cervical spinal cord as well as numerous cranial and cervical nerves, including the brachial plexus. Sensation to the neck itself is supplied by the cervical plexus derived from the ventral roots of C2, C3, C4, and occasionally C1. The vascular, lymphatic, and neurologic structures in the neck exhibit wide individual variation.

The thyroid gland, normally situated in the front of the lower part of the neck, consists of two lobes connected by a narrow isthmus. The lobes lie on the anterolateral aspect of the thyroid, cricoid, and upper tracheal cartilage. Occasionally a midline pyramidal lobe will be found between the two lateral lobes. Paired superior and inferior parathyroid glands are commonly seen on the undersurface of their respective thyroid lobes.

PHYSIOLOGY

Support

The cervical spine and its associated paraspinal muscles support and stabilize the head on the rest of the body. Any trauma, infection, or neoplastic process affecting these structures will interfere with this function. The trapezius and sternocleidomastoid muscles, while providing some support to the head, are mainly responsible for the ability of the head to move and turn.

Conduit

The triad of the larynx, trachea, and esophagus make the neck a conduit for respiration and alimentation. The carotid and vertebral arterial systems carry blood to the head and face, while the jugular system drains these same areas. The cervical spinal cord and several cervical and cranial nerves pass through the neck on their way to their ultimate destinations. A vast network of lymphatic channels serves to drain the areas of the head, face, and neck into the main lymph channels of the torso.

METHODS OF EXAMINATION

Direct Examination

Visual inspection and palpation provide the basis for examination of the neck and its enclosed structures. The subject's head should be erect on the neck and the neck symmetrical with normal prominence of the sterno-cleidomastoid muscle on each side. The anterior projection of the thyroid cartilage, or Adam's apple, is present in postpubescent males.

Congenital sinus tracts and neck masses can often be seen on direct examination. A neck mass that increases in size with crying or straining may indicate a vascular origin. Palpation of the neck is performed to determine both the size and consistency of the sternocleidomastoid muscles and the presence and nature of any cervical masses. Each side should be examined simultaneously so that one can be compared with the other. The examiner should be able to grasp the thyroid cartilage and move it gently from side to side without causing discomfort to the patient. Crepitance of the neck indicates the presence of free air in the tissue planes of the neck, as would result from perforation of a hollow viscus. Passive and active range of motion of the neck should be complete in all directions. Restricted movement may be the result of tender cervical adenopathy, cervical spine disease, spasm or fibrosis of the sternocleidomastoid muscle, or meningeal irritation. Arterial pulses should be palpated over the carotid artery on each side of the neck. The carotids can also be auscultated for evidence of bruits.

Radiologic Examination

Radiographs are often an invaluable aid in examination of the neck. Plain anterior-posterior and lateral views provide significant information in the evaluation of cervical problems. For example, masses projecting into and compromising the airway can be detected. The presence of air between the muscle planes of the neck indicates the perforation of a hollow viscus such as the pharynx, esophagus, larynx, trachea, or bronchus. Magnetic resonance (MR) imaging or computed tomography (CT) scans provide even finer detail of the neck. Ultrasound scans can be used to determine the solid or cystic nature of a cervical mass. Thyroid scans are helpful not only in evaluating the thyroid gland, but in confirming the presence of a thyroglossal duct cyst or ectopic thyroid tissue. If a mass is suspected to be of salivary gland origin, sialography will provide a detailed picture of the salivary duct system and will show the size and location of the gland itself.

Endoscopy

Any cervical condition suspected of being related to one or more of the hollow viscera that traverse the neck, such as the larynx, esophagus, or trachea should be evaluated endoscopically (by laryngoscopy, esophagoscopy, or bronchoscopy, respectively). These procedures usually require a general anesthesia and should be performed by an otolaryngologist.

Electrodiagnostic Tests

Electrodiagnostic tests are often helpful in evaluating such conditions as cranial or peripheral nerve palsies and primary muscle diseases. These studies include electromyograms and nerve conduction and excitability tests.

COMMON COMPLAINTS

Stiff Neck

Stiff neck also known as *wryneck* or *torticollis*, is an acute or chronic condition in which an abnormal contraction of some of the cervical muscles twists the neck into an unnatural position. The etiology of this condition is usually evident upon careful physical examination of the cervical structures. The most common cause of wryneck in a child is *tender cervical adenopathy*, related to an infection of the head and neck. Tender, enlarged lymph nodes lying between the sternocleidomastoid muscle and the deeper paraspinal muscles supporting the head can often be palpated. Motion of the head and neck can cause pressure on acutely swollen lymph nodes in the neck. By flexing and maintaining the neck to one side or the other, the child is able to minimize pressure on these tender nodes and reduce the amount of pain. Treatment of the primary infection and of the associated adenopathy with antibiotics will resolve the torticollis.

Trauma to the sternocleidomastoid muscle can cause an acute sprain and concomitant pain in the muscle. The neck is usually held flexed toward the side of injury in an effort to minimize stretching the injured muscle. The muscle is tender to palpation and contracted as compared with the normal side. Therapy, consisting of heat, oral analgesics, and rest, followed by range-of-motion exercises (once the initial injury has subsided), will usually induce complete resolution of the problem. A cervical collar may be helpful in some cases.

Meningeal irritation is another cause of wryneck. Flexion of the neck will produce tension in the inflamed meninges, reflexively activating the neck extensors to immobilize the cervical spine. The child reacts by resisting flexion of the neck, as will be indicated during physical examination.

Two rather uncommon congenital causes of torticollis are the *sternocleidomastoid tumor of infancy* and *congenital absence of the sternocleidomastoid muscle*. The sternocleidomastoid tumor of infancy is not a true neoplasm but is actually the result of fibrosis of the sternocleidomastoid muscle following perinatal trauma and hematoma formation. A firm mass is often palpable within the substance of the sternocleidomastoid muscle in a three- to four-week-old infant. (See the section on neoplasms, below, for further discussion of this condition.) Congenital absence of the sternocleidomastoid muscle is a rare cause of wryneck. The diagnosis is usually evident upon physical examination.

Some investigators hold that vestibular or ocular pathology can be a cause of torticollis. According to this theory, since vestibular or visual disturbances can cause vertigo or blurred vision with the head in the upright or neutral position, flexing the neck to one side can neutralize these sensory imbalances. The child learns to keep the head flexed to that side in order to keep the image of the environment both steady and clear. This compensatory position, however, eventually results in torticollis. Tempting though this connection may be, only a few cases of *vestibular* or *ocular torticollis* have been well documented, and the existence of these entities is still controversial.

Neck Mass

A wide variety of local and systemic etiologies are responsible for the appearance of a neck mass in a child (see Table 5-1). *Inflamed cervical lymph nodes* account for most neck masses in children. Recurrent viral or bacterial infections of the upper aerodigestive tract (including ears, nose, sinus, pharynx, larynx, and oral cavity), the thyroid gland, and the skin of the head and neck can also cause acute or chronic enlargement of cervical lymph nodes. The acutely enlarged masses are usually distinguished by a history of an associated febrile illness with symptoms referable to the primary infection, such as an ear infection or tonsillitis. The nodes are often multiple and tender to palpation. The skin overlying the lesions is often erythematous and warm to the touch. An abscess in the nodes is indicated by fluctuance and by the shiny-red thin appearance of the overlying skin.

Enlarged lymph nodes related to chronic or recurrent infections are also usually multiple, but other signs of acute inflammation are absent. These discrete nodes are firm and mobile but nontender to palpation. A history of multiple infections of the head and neck helps identify the etiology of the neck mass. Chronically infected lymph nodes secondary to bacterial, viral, acquired toxoplasmosis, and cat-scratch infections are indistinguishable on the basis of physical examination alone. Laboratory studies such as serum titer, culture of aspirate, or biopsy for histologic examination are often necessary to identify the pathogenic organism.

Another common category of neck masses in children is that related to *congenital causes*. While some of these masses might not become apparent until the child is several years of age, all are considered congenital in nature. *Branchial cleft cysts* usually appear in the lateral neck, anterior to the sternocleidomastoid muscle, and deep to the platysma muscle. Their cystic nature is often detectable upon physical examination. A sinus tract

Table 5-1   Causes of Neck Masses in Children

Congenital
   Branchial cleft cysts
   Thyroglossal duct remnants
   Laryngocele
   Ectopic thyroid
   Lymphangioma (cystic hygroma)
Inflammatory (lymph node, salivary gland)
   Bacteria
   Virus
   Fungus
   Parasite
   Mycobacteria
      tuberculosis
      Atypical
   Miscellaneous
      Sarcoid
      Cat scratch
      Mucocutaneous lymph node (Kawasaki)
Metabolic
   Dilantin (diphenyhydantoin)
   Hyperthyroidism (goiter)
Traumatic
   Hematoma
   Arteriovenous fistula
   Sternocleidomastoid "tumor" of infancy
Neoplastic
   Benign
   Malignant
      Primary (usually mesenchymal)
      Metastatic

---

may be present connecting the cyst to the overlying neck skin. *Thyroglossal duct cysts* classically present in the midline of the neck at the level of the hyoid bone. The examiner will note that the mass moves up and down with swallowing and protrusion of the tongue. *Laryngoceles* are uncommon lesions in children. These congenital dilations of the laryngeal ventricle extend through the cricothyroid membrane, presenting laterally in the neck. Crepitance is often detected during palpation of the cystic mass, as laryngoceles may contain air. Ultrasound or radiography will confirm the diagnosis.

A *hemangioma* is a congenital vascular malformation. The diagnosis is usually evident upon physical examination of a red to reddish-purple lesion that blanches with pressure. In a subcutaneous hemangioma, the bluish discoloration of the skin may be absent, complicating the diagnosis. The examiner should be attentive to a possible bruit heard over the mass, enlargement with crying or straining, and the presence of other cutaneous hemangiomas in order to confirm the diagnosis of hemangiomas in the neck.

Lymphangioma, or *cystic hygroma*, is a congenital lesion of lymphatic tissue. It usually presents as a large, fluctuant, lateral neck mass that transilluminates. Lymphangiomas may fluctuate in size in association with lymphadenitis, related to an infection of the head and neck.

Trauma can be the cause of several different types of neck mass. *Acute hematoma* will usually present with a rather diffuse swelling and tenderness. Often, the skin overlying the mass has a bluish discoloration. The *sternocleidomastoid tumor of infancy* is not really a tumor, but the result of perinatal trauma. (It is discussed in detail in the section on trauma — *see* page 164.) *Traumatic arteriovenous fistulas* will not appear until several weeks after cervical trauma. A mass, often pulsatile, will be found at the site of the previous injury. Auscultation of the mass will demonstrate a bruit, and an angiogram or MRA will confirm the diagnosis.

Lymphoma is the most common malignancy of the head and neck in children. The cervical mass may be either a primary lesion or a metastasis from a primary lesion in the mouth or pharynx. The nodes are multiple, matted together, and rubbery-firm in consistency and may be either unilateral or bilateral. Other malignant lesions that present in the neck of children include *rhabdomyosarcoma, neuroblastoma, squamous cell carcinoma of the nasopharynx, salivary gland malignancy* and *thyroid malignancy.* These malignant lesions are not easily distinguished, as there is little in the clinical appearance of the neck mass to differentiate them. The masses are usually singular, but may be multiple, and are firm to hard in nature. They may be fixed to surrounding structures. Any neck mass that is suspicious of malignancy requires a complete examination of the head and neck, radiographs (possibly including CT or MR scan), and ultimately, a biopsy. The presence of an associated finding in the head and neck, such as a thyroid mass or sinus destruction on sinus radiographs, would be useful in identifying the nature of the cervical mass.

Another group of lesions that present in the neck are secondary to a drug reaction or to a *metabolic abnormality*. Diphenylhydantoin (Dilantin), for example, can cause benign cervical adenopathy (in addition to the more commonly seen gingival hypertrophy); when the drug is stopped, the lesion generally regresses. Rare cases of lymphoma or pseudolymphoma have been reported as well. Mesantoin (mephenytoin) can cause lymphadenopathy that mimics Hodgkin's disease. The clinical presentation is identical to that associated with adenopathy of infectious or neoplastic origin.

Thyroid enlargement related to *hyperthyroidism* presents with a diffusely enlarged, nontender thyroid gland in a child exhibiting the usual symptoms of hyperthyroidism (e.g., tremor, excessive perspiration, emotional lability, tachycardia, increased basal metabolism, goiter). Likewise, subacute inflammation of the thyroid gland, thyroiditis, causes enlargement and tenderness. Localized masses within the thyroid gland may be result of thyroid cysts, functioning and non-functioning thyroid nodules and rarely, malignant tumors.

Swelling of the parotid glands may be seen in adolescents with bulemia. Submandibular gland enlargement is frequently seen in children with cystic fibrosis. The parotid gland is less involved in those patients due to the lesser number of mucous glands in the parotid compared to the submandibular glands.

Several disease entities of unknown etiology often have associated lymph node enlargement. *Sarcoidosis* is a disorder characterized by granulomas that can affect the reticuloendothelial system, respiratory tract, eye, and central nervous system. The diagnosis is suspected on the basis of the clinical presentation and is confirmed by the demonstration of noncaseating granulomas on a biopsy of a minor salivary gland, tracheal mucosa (or transbronchial lung parenchyma), or on enlarged cervical or mediastinal lymph nodes. *Mucocutaneous lymph node syndrome (Kawasaki's disease)* is an idiopathic disorder distinguished by cervical adenopathy, fever, bilateral conjunctival injection, mucous membrane changes, rash, erythema and/or scaling of the extremities, and occasional cardiac abnormalities. No specific laboratory tests or histologic findings have been found helpful in confirming the diagnosis of this syndrome. The diagnosis is confirmed clinically by the presence of five or six major criteria.

As can be seen from the great variety of causes of head and neck masses, the presence of a cervical mass in a child necessitates a complete workup to determine the etiology. A thorough history (including perinatal events) and complete examination of the head and neck are the first steps in the evaluation. Careful examination of the nose, mouth, pharynx, and larynx is warranted if indicated by the history or symptoms. Radiographs of the neck, sinuses, skull, or mandible may be necessary, depending on the specific characteristics. Blood studies may be helpful, especially if the lesion is suspected to be of thyroid origin or related to a drug reaction. Serum titers (viral, bacterial) are useful in evaluating neck masses of suspected inflammatory origin. Elevated titers to the Epstein-Barr virus are associated with Burkitt's lymphoma and squamous cell carcinoma of the nasopharynx.

Often the maneuvers described above will identify the cause of the neck mass, and the appropriate treatment — medical or surgical — can be instituted. If, however, the diagnosis is still unknown, surgical intervention will be necessary for diagnostic and therapeutic purposes. If possible, excisional biopsy is preferable to incisional biopsy. It has the advantages of removing the entire lesion, thereby presenting a larger specimen to the pathologist, and of avoiding spillage of a possible neoplastic process. Once the diagnosis of the neck mass has been obtained, further evaluation and treatment can begin.

CONGENITAL MALFORMATIONS

Branchial Cleft Anomalies

The four-week-old embryo has five epithelia-lined ridges projecting laterally from each side of the pharynx. These pharyngeal or branchial arches are separated by branchial clefts — the forerunners of the gill system of fish. Each of the arches is associated with its own neural, arterial, and cartilaginous structure. As the embryo continues to develop, the arches coalesce to obliterate the clefts. Persistence of a cleft leads to branchial cleft anomalies in the neck. The nature of the anomaly depends on the degree of obliteration of the branchial clefts and the stage of differentiation of its cartilaginous structures. If the lateral aspect of the cleft has been obliterated, the epithelial-lined space will form a cyst. Persistent communication to the pharynx or to the neck skin will convert this cyst into a sinus tract. If the cyst communicates to both the skin and pharynx, a fistula will form. Portions of lymphoid tissue and cartilage rests associated with the particular branchial arch involved may also be present within or near the malformation.

Because the epithelial ridge that forms the lower border of the branchial arches contains material destined to become the sternocleidomastoid muscle and the hypoglossal nerve, all branchial cleft anomalies must present (or pass) in an anterior-superior direction relative to these structures. This detail is not only helpful in making the clinical diagnosis of the anomaly, but is also crucial to subsequent surgical treatment as well. Identification of the nerves, arteries, and cartilage derivatives associated with the branchial cleft malformation will enable the surgeon to determine the origin of the anomaly (i.e., first cleft, second cleft) and will assist in the surgical dissection.

Branchial cleft cysts present as soft, cystic masses anterior to the sternocleidomastoid muscle. Although congenital in origin, these anomalies rarely present in the newborn infant. While the pit of a sinus tract may be apparent at birth, symptomatic enlargement or presentation of a mass usually does not occur until the child is older. It may take several months or even years for a cyst to accumulate sufficient epithelial debris or secretions to present as a mass lesion. If the contents of the cyst (or the associated lymphoid tissue) become infected, the child will present with an acutely swollen, tender neck mass. In the case of a sinus tract, drainage onto the neck or into the pharynx may occur.

Anomalies of the first branchial cleft are uncommon. They occur in proximity to the external auditory canal, also a derivative of the first and second branchial arches surrounding the first branchial cleft. These lesions may present as a swollen, tender cystic mass inferior or posterior to the lobule of the ear. If the cyst communicates with the external ear canal, pressure applied to the mass will provide purulent material in the external meatus. The lesion must be differentiated clinically from the much more common and superficial sebaceous cyst. A sinus tract is frequently located near the facial nerve, or even between its branches.

Anomalies of the second branchial cleft present laterally in the neck, deep to the platysma, and anterior to the sternocleidomastoid muscle. A sinus tract, if present, would have to pass superior to the hypoglossal nerve, inferior to the glossopharyngeal nerve (nerve of the third branchial arch) and between the internal and external branches of the carotid artery to terminate in the area of the faucial tonsils. (The faucial tonsils are derivatives of the second and third arches surrounding the second cleft or pouch.)

Anomalies of the third branchial cleft, while probably less common than those of the second cleft, present in a similar manner. The sinus tract of the third branchial cleft, if present, is differentiated from that of the second branchial cleft by its course below the glossopharyngeal nerve and posterior to both branches of the glossopharyngeal nerve and posterior to both branches of the carotid artery, whereupon it enters the pharynx in the area of the pyriform sinus. (The pyriform sinus is formed by the third and fourth branchial arches surrounding the third branchial cleft or pouch. Fourth branchial cleft anomalies appear to be only theoretical possibilities, since none have been reported.)

If a branchial cleft anomaly is suspected, a complete examination of the head and neck, including the oral cavity and pharynx, should be performed. Referral should be made to an otolaryngologist to assist the primary practitioner in the workup, as failure to identify all the aspects of the anomaly may lead to an incorrect diagnosis and inappropriate treatment. Radiographs, specifically CT or MR scans, of the head and neck may be helpful in evaluating these malformations. Ultrasound can determine whether the lesion is cystic, separating it from solid lesions such as lymph nodes and neoplastic lesions of the neck. If a sinus tract is present, a radiopaque dye can be gently injected to visualize the lesion and its extensions.

Proper treatment of branchial cleft anomalies involves complete excision of all epithelial-lined remnants without sacrifice of any vital structure. Incomplete removal of the branchial cleft anomaly will only lead to recurrence and the necessity of secondary surgery in a scarred area. The carotid arteries, facial nerve, and pharynx may be intimately involved with the lesion, and they should be identified and preserved.

Thyroid Malformations

The thyroid gland is derived from the second branchial arch and originates at the foramen cecum of the base of the tongue. During the second month of fetal life, the gland begins its descent in the neck. The tissue passes through the substance of the tongue, courses near or through the hyoid bone, and comes to rest in its normal anterior and lateral to the thyroid cartilage. Generally, no sign of this developmental descent remains in the infant. Occasionally, however, incomplete descent of the gland or persistence of the thyroglossal duct occurs as a congenital anomaly.

Ectopic Thyroid

Ectopic thyroid tissue is any thyroid tissue that occurs outside its normal position. Aberrant tissue may occur anywhere in the neck , but the most common sites are along the path of the normal descent of the gland. The abnormality is termed *lingual* or *cervical thyroid,* depending upon the location of the aberrant tissue. Ectopic thyroid has only rarely been found within the esophagus or trachea. While some authorities contend that

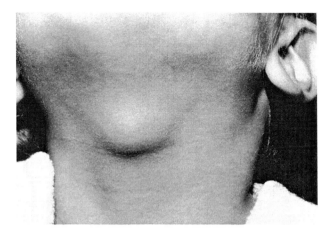

Figure 5–2. Thyroglossal duct cyst presenting as a midline neck mass at the level of the hyoid bone.

ectopic thyroid tissue can occur laterally in the neck, most investigators believe that the tissue is more likely a metastatic thyroid carcinoma. Biopsy of the suspected ectopic thyroid mass and thyroid gland may be necessary to differentiate ectopic thyroid tissue from metastatic thyroid neoplasm, since both entities will demonstrate uptake of radioactive iodine (^{131}I) on a thyroid scan.

Once a diagnosis of ectopic thyroid has been made, no further treatment is required unless other symptoms are present. For example, obstruction of the airway by a lingual or tracheal thyroid will require emergency surgical excision. Even when left in place, ectopic thyroid tissue may fail to produce thyroid hormone at some later date. For this reason, the child's thyroid function should be carefully monitored at frequent follow-up visits. If the child begins to demonstrate signs and symptoms of hypothyroidism (e.g., decreased growth velocity, constipation, decreased basal metabolic rate, lethargy, sensitivity to cold), treatment with exogenous thyroid should be begun.

Thyroglossal Duct Remnants

Epithelial rests that persist along the course of the descent of the thyroid gland will result in the formation of thyroglossal duct anomalies. A midline neck cyst at or below the level of the hyoid bone is the most common example of this problem (Fig. 5-2). Because the malformation is often connected to the tongue above and the thyroid gland (adherent to the thyroid cartilage) below, the cyst moves up and down with protrusion of the tongue and with deglutition. The cyst grows slowly as a result of accumulated mucoid material within the epithelial-lined cyst. Sudden growth is usually indicative of infection. Since there is no embryonic connection between the cyst and the overlying skin of the neck, drainage to the anterior neck can only result from previous needle aspiration, incision and drainage or incomplete removal of the cyst. The differential diagnosis includes other masses that can present in the midline of the neck such as lymph nodes lesions, dermoid cysts, ectopic thyroid, and various neoplasms.

If a thyroglossal duct or cyst is suspected, ultrasound of the neck can confirm the presence of a normal thyroid gland. This is done to determine whether there is functioning thyroid tissue separate from the anomaly. This information is crucial to a discussion with the parents concerning the proposed treatment and possible risk of hypothyroidism. Surgical excision is the treatment of choice for thyroglossal duct/cyst remnants, because this procedure confirms the diagnosis, prevents recurrent infections, and rules out other, more serious entities. Careful surgical dissection and removal of all epithelial remnants is required to prevent recurrence of the anomaly. Because the descent of the thyroid may leave one or more epithelial tracts coursing near or even through the hyoid bone, the central portion of the hyoid bone is removed along with the surgical specimen (Sistrunk operation) to ensure complete removal of all epithelial-lined structures.

Hemangiomas and Lymphangiomas

The *hemangioma* is the most common congenital malformation of the head and neck in children. It has been estimated that up to 10% of all children have some type of hemangioma at, or shortly after, birth. Although more common on the skin of the face and scalp, these vascular malformations can occur on the skin of the neck and involve deeper structures such as the parotid gland. The diagnosis of cutaneous hemangiomas of the cervical skin is usually obvious upon by physical inspection; the lesions are red to reddish-purple and flat or raised; they blanch with pressure and increase in size with crying or straining. The vascular nature of deep-seated lesions can be demonstrated on MR with contrast.

Juvenile hemangiomas demonstrate a cycle of rapid growth for the first 12 to 18 months of life followed by slow regression and even total disappearance over the next year or two. Because of this natural history, the preferred treatment is close observation. Lesions that grow rapidly and that produce complications, such as airway obstruction, hemorrhage, high-output cardiac failure, or thrombocytopenia clearly require active intervention. Corticosteroids (prednisone 1 mg/kg-day for two weeks) are highly effective in halting the growth of hemangiomas and may even induce early resolution. Cryotherapy, laser excision, and sclerosing agents have all been used to treat rapidly enlarging lesions, but these methods have significant limitations with respect to the size and location of the hemangioma that can be treated and to such considerations as the resultant scar. Attempts at surgical excision carry the potential for life-threatening hemorrhage and usually only result in partial resection of the lesion. While radiation therapy can be successful in shrinking hemangiomas, the carcinogenic potential of this mode of therapy makes it an undesirable method of treatment of such a benign disorder. Lesions that demonstrate cosmetic or functional disability after incomplete resolution may be considered possible candidates for surgical excision.

Lymphangiomas are congenital malformations of lymphatic tissue. Some investigators classify lymphangiomas on the basis of histologic appearance: lymphangioma simplex, cavernous lymphangioma, and cystic hygroma. Cystic hygroma is the most common type of lymphangioma found in the neck. These lesions consist of multiple cystic spaces filled with lymph and, occasionally, blood. They present most commonly as large lateral neck masses in neonates and infants. The diagnosis is often obvious upon physical examination of a large cystic lesion that transilluminates. The natural history of these lesions is usually one of progressive growth and enlargement. These lesions can fluctuate in size secondary to a concurrent infection of the head and neck or hemorrhage into a cyst. There is no predictable regression of lymphangiomas, as seen in hemangiomas.

Small, stable, asymptomatic lesions can probably be managed by close observation and surgery only if symptoms related to the mass occur. Surgical excision is the treatment of choice for all other lesions, with several staged procedures often required. The infiltrative nature of a cystic hygroma requires meticulous dissection with attention to sparing vital neural and vascular structures in the neck. Aspiration of a large cyst can temporarily decompress a lesion, but this technique is not a substitute for definitive surgical excision. Large cystic hygromas can cause feeding difficulties or respiratory distress in the newborn, necessitating early surgical intervention; tracheostomy and gastrostomy may be required as well.

INFECTIOUS DISEASES

Cervical Adenitis

Cervical adenitis is the most common cause of a neck mass in a child. The lymphatic system of the neck drains the internal cavities of the head and neck (ear, eye, nose, mouth, pharynx, sinuses, larynx) as well as the thyroid, skin, and associated adnexal structures of the face and scalp. A primary infection of any of these will lead to involvement of the regional cervical lymph nodes. Since certain groups of nodes drain specific sites in the head and neck, the location of the swollen and infected lymph node often helps the practitioner in identifying the area of the primary infection (Fig. 5-3). Ear infections most often drain to the pre-, post-, and infra-auricular nodes. Pharyngeal infections (e.g., tonsillitis) usually present with jugulodigastric node involvement. Enlarged posterior cervical nodes often accompany nasopharyngeal infections (e.g., adenoiditis).

The organism responsible for the cervical adenopathy is usually the same organism that has caused the primary infection. Cervical adenopathy is uncommon secondary to the brief, uncomplicated, viral upper respiratory infection. Enlarged nodes occur more commonly as a result of bacterial infection of the head and neck, particularly of the ears and pharynx. Since streptococcal species account for most bacterial infections in the head and neck, the infected lymph nodes will contain the same organisms. Treatment with oral penicillin (or ampicillin) usually clears the primary infection and brings about regression of the enlarged lymph nodes.

Although most cases will respond to penicillin therapy, a small group of children will be found in whom the enlarged lymph nodes will not regress; these resistant cases require further treatment. Studies of children hospitalized with cervical adenitis have shown a predominance of *Staphylococcus aureus* as the causative agent. This high incidence of *Staphylococcus* is probably the result of selecting out patients who have not responded to a course of oral antimicrobials usually prescribed against the more commonly occurring *Streptococcus* species. Therefore, if a child has not responded to the primary antimicrobial treatment, agents should be added that are known to be effective against *Staphylococcus aureus*, such as erythromycin, dicloxacillin, and the cephalosporins.

A child who is found to have rapid enlargement of cervical nodes, cellulitis of the overlying skin, abscess formation, or signs of toxicity (high fever, malaise, dehydration) should be admitted to the hospital for treatment with

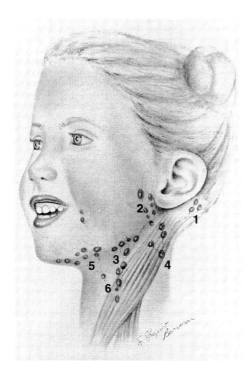

Figure 5–3. Lymphatic drainage of the head and neck.

1 = Post-auricular	4 = Posterior cervical
2 = Pre-auricular	5 = Submandibular
3 = Jugulo-digastric	6 = Anterior cervical

intravenous fluids and antimicrobials. If fluctuance is present, aspiration can be performed to decompress the node and to provide material for culture and antibiotic sensitivity. If there is no evidence of fluctuance, 1 ml of sterile saline (nonbacteriostatic) can be injected into the node and then aspirated back for the same purpose.

While formal incision and drainage of an abscess can hasten obliteration of the abscess cavity, repeated needle aspiration serves the same purpose and avoids a surgical scar. The application of heat to the affected nodes can provide some comfort as well as hasten resolution of the process. Once the infection begins to resolve and the child no longer demonstrates signs of toxicity, a course of oral antimicrobials may be instituted and continued on an outpatient basis for a full 10 to 14 days.

If the cervical adenopathy does not respond after the above regimen, further intervention is indicated for diagnostic and therapeutic purposes. If the practitioner feels confident that the enlarged lymph nodes are secondary to chronic or recurrent inflammatory disease of the head and neck, such as tonsillitis or otitis, definitive treatment of these conditions may be curative.

Neck nodes that continue to drain after aspiration or incision and drainage may be caused by an unusual organism for the site. Complete excision of the node and sinus tracts if often required for diagnosis and treatment. Biopsy and excision of the cervical node are indicated to rule out neoplasm and other sources of infection. *Mycobacterium* (*tuberculosis* and atypical), *Toxoplasma gondii, Actinomyces iraelii*, and other organisms are among the uncommon causes of cervical adenopathy. Cat scratch disease is another rare cause of enlarged cervical nodes in children. Once the diagnosis of these infections has been made, specific therapy can be directed toward the causative agent.

Retropharyngeal or parapharyngeal nodes are often involved with inflammatory processes that originate in the pharynx, but these nodes rarely present with clinically significant symptoms. Sore throat, dysphagia, and stiff neck are some of the symptoms that can accompany markedly enlarged pharyngeal nodes. Enlarged retropharyngeal nodes can be detected overlying the cervical spine during examination of the oropharynx. They also appear as a bulge or widening of the retropharyngeal soft tissues on lateral neck radiographs. Inflamed parapharyngeal nodes are seldom detected clinically unless they enlarge sufficiently to deviate the tonsil and pharyngeal wall medially. Treatment of enlarged pharyngeal nodes consists of intravenous administration of antibiotics, careful observation for possible airway obstruction, and biopsy if resolution does not occur with treatment or if a malignancy is suspected. If airway obstruction occurs, intervention with intubation, abscess drainage, and possibly tracheotomy, is required.

Neck Abscess

A collection of purulent material within the tissues of the neck requires prompt and specific treatment. The most common cause of a neck abscess is the breakdown or necrosis of an infected lymph node. Purulent material may be located within a single node or may accumulate between several adjacent nodes. Once the process of cervical adenitis has progressed to the point of abscess formation, treatment is directed toward evacuation of the infected material and prevention of the further spread of infection. The child is hospitalized and intravenous antimicrobials effective against *Staphylococcus aureus* are administered. Needle aspiration or formal incision and drainage can be used to evacuate the infected material. Again, the former method may require multiple aspirations, but it is the favored treatment because it eliminates the need for a large incision (and resultant scar) and for the general anesthetic usually required to perform a formal incision and drainage of a neck abscess in a child.

Deep neck abscesses are uncommon in children but can be extremely dangerous when they occur. *Parapharyngeal abscess* occurs when purulent material collects in the parapharyngeal space lateral to the pharyngeal constrictors and medial to the vascular compartment of the neck. Necrosis of parapharyngeal lymph nodes and lateral extension of a peritonsillar abscess are the two main sources of this infection. The child presents with a stiff neck, high fever, malaise, dehydration, and other signs of toxicity. He usually has dysphagia for solids and may not be able to swallow his own saliva. Physical examination reveals diffuse swelling and tenderness on one side of the neck, but fluctuance is seldom appreciated. Intraoral examination may demonstrate medial displacement of the lateral pharyngeal wall and its faucial tonsil. While lateral neck radiographs are usually not helpful in evaluating this disease process, a CT scan can often demonstrate the soft tissue swelling and mass effect of the abscess. If left to progress, the parapharyngeal abscess could involve the adjacent vascular structures in the neck, descend into the pharynx and cause aspiration or asphyxiation. Appropriate treatment consists of hospitalization and administration of intravenous fluids and antimicrobials effective against *Staphylococcus aureus*. After 12 to 24 hours of intravenous hydration and antimicrobial therapy, the signs of toxicity will have decreased; the abscess should then be drained through an external neck incision. Resolution of the process occurs quickly with this regimen.

Retropharyngeal abscess occurs as a result of the necrosis of retropharyngeal lymph nodes or secondary to perforation of the pharynx or esophagus. Purulent material collects between the retropharyngeal and prevertebral layers of the cervical fascia, also known as the *danger space*. This potential space extends from the base of the skull to mediastinum, allowing for extensive spread of the infection. Presenting symptoms are similar to these associated with parapharyngeal abscess. Lateral neck radiographs will demonstrate widening and bulging of the retropharyngeal space (see Fig. 3-2). Computed tomography is essential in distinguishing an abscess from just enlarged retropharyngeal lymph nodes. Treatment consists of hospitalization and a course of intravenous fluids and antimicrobials effective against *Staphylococcus aureus*. After 12 to 24 hours of intravenous antimicrobial therapy, drainage of the abscess should be performed through either an intraoral or an external neck incision.

Salivary Gland Infections

Salivary gland infections should be considered in the differential diagnosis of a cervical mass suspected of being infectious in origin. Both viral and bacterial agents can be responsible for the infection, with the former being much more common. Mumps (endemic parotitis) is the most common salivary infection in children. Other viral agents associated with parotitis include Coxsackie A, parainfluenzae, cytomegalovirus, and the Epstein-Barr virus. While the parotid gland is affected in more than 85% of cases, the submandibular gland may be involved as well. The infection presents with acute painful swelling of the involved gland or glands. Minimal erythema is seen around the intraoral orifice of the salivary duct, and the saliva expressed is generally clear. Treatment is symptomatic with clear fluids, antipyretics, and analgesics as necessary.

Bacterial infections of the salivary glands will present with signs and symptoms similar to those associated with cervical lymphadenitis. Neonatal parotitis and, less commonly, submandibular sialadenitis usually occur in a three- to four-week-old infant in whom a systemic illness has resulted in dehydration. Massage of the affected salivary gland may demonstrate expression of purulent material from either Stensen's or Wharton's duct. The affected gland is very swollen, and abscess formation may occur. Treatment consists of intravenous antimicrobials effective against *Staphylococcus aureus* and evacuation of any collection of purulent material.

Recurrent or chronic infections of the salivary glands are usually related to some predisposing factor. A ductal stricture, salivary gland stone, immune-deficiency state including that associated with HIV infection, or autoimmune disorder may be the underlying cause of periodic attacks of salivary gland inflammation. Once the acute infection has been treated, the child with recurrent infections should be further examined for signs of predisposing factors. Treatment should then be directed toward correction of these conditions. Such measures as disruption of the neural innervation of the salivary gland, salivary duct ligation, or even salivary gland excision may be required in the management of these difficult problems.

NEOPLASMS

Benign Neoplasms

Hemangiomas and *lymphangiomas* of the neck are benign masses that actually represent congenital malformations rather than true neoplasms. As such, they have been included and discussed on page 156.

Less common benign neoplasms of the neck in children include *teratomas, paragangliomas (carotid body tumors, glomus tumors), thyroid tumors,* and *salivary gland neoplasms.* Once the specific diagnosis has been made, treatment is begun appropriate to the nature and extent of the lesion.

Malignant Neoplasms

The most common malignant neoplasm of the neck in children is *lymphoma,* almost equally divided into *Hodgkin's* and *non-Hodgkin's* types. The disease may be localized in the neck or be a part of a more generalized disorder. Physical examination will often reveal multiple firm, rubbery, unilateral or bilateral nodes. If the diagnosis of lymphoma is suspected, an otolaryngologist should be consulted to perform a careful examination of the oral cavity, pharynx and paranasal sinuses, looking for a primary or associated lesion. This approach not only aids in the evaluation of the extent of the lesion, but may also serve to locate a site from which a biopsy can be obtained without the morbidity associated with a neck exploration. If biopsy of a neck node is required for diagnosis, the biopsy should be excisional to provide the pathologist with a complete lymph nodes for evaluation. The treatment of lymphoma depends upon the classification and stage at the time of diagnosis; radiation therapy is generally given for a localized disease, with the addition of chemotherapy for systemic or more diffuse involvement. Prognosis is also correlated with the classification and stage of the lymphoma at presentation. Cure rates are excellent in the more localized and well-differentiated forms of Hodgkin's disease; non-Hodgkin's lymphomas tend to be more disseminated and carry a poorer prognosis.

Rhabdomyosarcoma is the most common soft tissue sarcoma of the head and neck in children; its frequency of occurrence in the neck is second only to that in the orbit. The child will usually present with a history and physical examination, a biopsy is usually required for confirmation. The infiltrative nature and tendency toward early dissemination for these neoplasms seldom permit complete surgical excision. For this reason, the current treatment of rhabdomyosarcoma consists of radiation therapy and chemotherapy. Cure rates have improved significantly since the institution of aggressive therapy in the 1960s.

Cervical lymph modes may present with neoplasms that have metastasized from a nonlymphogenous primary. Squamous carcinoma of the nasopharynx, malignant melanoma, malignant fibrous histiocytoma, neuroblastoma, and thyroid or salivary gland malignancies may all present first with enlarged cervical lymph nodes. These nodes tend to be hard and singular and may be fixed to underlying structures. Otolaryngologic consultation should be obtained to perform a complete examination of the head and neck to search for a primary lesion. Biopsy of the node is usually required for diagnosis. Once again, excisional biopsy is recommended to present the pathologist with the most complete material form which to determine the diagnosis. Treatment and prognosis depend on the nature and extent of the neoplasm.

TRAUMA

Neck trauma can be an isolated injury or only one factor in a multisystem insult. In evaluating trauma of the neck, the physician should search for evidence of associated injuries to the vertebral column, head, chest, and abdomen. Management of these potentially more serious injuries may take precedence over the treatment of the cervical trauma.

The injuries are usually divided into blunt and penetrating types. *Blunt trauma* is by far the most common type of injury of the neck. Vehicular accidents (automobile, motorcycle, bicycle) and sports-related activities account for most of these occurrences. A bruise or hematoma of the soft tissues of the neck is the most common blunt injury of the neck. A tear of a small blood vessel as a result of the trauma allows blood to extravasate and infiltrate adjacent soft tissues. A child who has sustained this type of injury will complain of pain and swelling in the affected area. A bluish discoloration of the overlying skin often is not present at the time of the acute injury but will appear one or two days later. These injuries are most often self-limited and will resolve spontaneously within several days. Heat and rest usually aid in the recovery process.

Severe blunt trauma can result in injuries requiring more involved care. A progressively enlarging neck mass following cervical trauma may indicate persistent hemorrhage from a large blood vessel. An angiogram or MRA (magnetic resonance angiography) followed by surgical exploration and ligation of the bleeding vessel is often required in these cases. The airway may become compromised in these patients, requiring endotracheal intubation or tracheostomy. Cranial nerve deficits indicate a serious injury of the deep tissues of the neck or base of skull and require careful neurologic evaluation with possible neck exploration. Blunt trauma to the anterior neck can result in laryngeal injury (see Chapter 4 for an in-depth discussion).

A possible late sequela of vascular injury is the arteriovenous fistula. The diagnosis is suggested by a pulsatile mass appearing several weeks after the injury. Surgical exploration and resection of the fistula is the treatment of choice.

Penetrating injuries of the neck pose many difficult problems both in evaluation and in management. Once again, severe associated injuries may required treatment first. The nature of the injury must be determined during the initial evaluation: length of knife, caliber of bullet, number of entrance and exit wounds, apparent course of missile, and so forth. As in all emergency cases, the status of the airway should be ascertained as the first priority. The presence of respiratory distress, stridor, hemoptysis, subcutaneous emphysema, or hoarseness can all indicate possible airway injury. Excessive hemorrhage, absent pulse, and expanding neck swelling are all signs of significant vascular injury. Compression of the bleeding site is the second emergency priority; an angiogram or MRA and surgical exploration may also play a role in the management of these injuries. While some investigators consider any laceration or penetrating injury deep to the platysma muscle cause for surgical intervention, most reserve surgical exploration for selective cases in which signs of symptoms of significant vascular or airway injury are demonstrated. A complete neurologic examination must be performed to detect any injuries to the spinal cord and cranial and other peripheral nerves. Otolaryngological consultation will include indirect and direct laryngoscopy and bronchoscopy as required to determine the presence and extent of damage to the larynx and trachea.

The *sternocleidomastoid tumor of infancy* is an uncommon cause of torticollis in the newborn. Not a neoplasm, this condition is though to be related to perinatal trauma. A significant proportion of these neonates have had a history of difficult labor, breech presentation, or difficult delivery (e.g., forceps). By contrast, some infants with this condition have been born by cesarean section and have had no identifiable cervical trauma during the pregnancy. Ultrasound studies have even demonstrated these presence of wryneck deformity in the developing fetus. The histopathology of this condition appears to start with a traumatic hematoma within the sternocleidomastoid muscle. The hematoma beings to organize, leading to fibrosis of the surrounding damaged muscle during the third or fourth week of life. At this time, a mass is noted within the substance of the sternocleidomastoid muscle. Management should be conservative because most of these lesions resolve without any further treatment. Heat and passive range-of-motion exercises are recommended to hasten resolution of the process and to prevent fibrotic shortening of the sternocleidomastoid muscle and resultant torticollis. If the lesion does not begin to recede after one to two months of conservative management, surgical exploration and biopsy may be necessary to confirm the diagnosis and to rule out other, potentially more dangerous lesions. If the fibrotic process progresses to cause a wryneck deformity, resection of the fibrous mass and lengthening of the sternocleidomastoid may be required at a later time.

SUGGESTED READINGS

Anderson GJ, Tom LWC, Womer RB, Handler SD, Wetmore RF, Potsic WP: Rhabdomyosarcoma of the head and neck in children. *Arch Otolaryngol Head Neck Surg* 116:428-431, 1990.

Bamji M, Stone R, Kaul A, Usmani G, Schachter F, Wasserman E: Palpable lymph nodes in healthy newborns and infants. *Pediatrics* 78:573-575, 1986.

Dodds B, Maniglia AJ: Peritonsillar and neck abscesses in the pediatric age group. *Laryngoscope* 98:956-959, 1988.

Garfinkle TS, Handler SD: Hemangiomas of the head and neck in children: Guide to management. *J Otolaryngol* 9:439-450, 1980.

Handler SD: Diagnosis and management of maxillo-facial injuries. In: Torg J (ed): Athletic Injuries to the Head and Neck. Philadelphia, Lea and Febiger. 1982, pp. 223-244.

Handler SD, Raney RB: Management of neoplasms of the head and neck in children. I. Benign tumors. *Head Neck Surg* 3:395-405, 1981.

Hawkins DB, Austin JR: Abscesses of the neck in infants and young children: A review of 112 cases. *Ann Otol Rhinol Laryngol* 100:361-365, 1991.

Herzog L: Prevalence of lymphadenopathy of the head and neck in children. *Clin Pediatr* 22:485-487, 1983.

Kennedy TL: Curettage of nontuberculous mycobacteria cervical lymphadenitis. *Arch Otolaryngol Head Neck Surg* 118:759-762, 1992.

Knight PJ, Mulne AF, Vassy LE: When is lymph node biopsy indicated in children with enlarged peripheral nodes? *Pediatrics* 69:391-396, 1982.

Raney RB, Handler SD: Management of neoplasms of head and neck in children. II. Malignant tumors. *Head Neck Surg* 3:500-507, 1981.

Tom LWC, Handler SD, Wetmore RF, Potsic WP: The sternocleidomastoid tumor of infancy. *Int J Pediatr Otorhinolaryngol* 13:245-255, 1987.

Torsiglieri AJ, Tom LWC, Ross AJ, Wetmore RF, Handler SD, Potsic WP: Pediatric neck masses: Guidelines for evaluation. *Int J Pediatr Otorhinolaryngol* 16:199-210, 1988.

Index